Cinderella Solution Your Complete System

Carly Donovan

Copyright © 2019 Carly Donovan

All rights reserved.

ISBN: 9781082346149

CONTENTS

1 PART ONE: THE CINDERELLA SOLUTION EXPLAINED — 1

2 PART TWO: MEAL CREATEOR & FLAVOR PAIRING — 38

3 PART THERE: Cinderella's TOP 10: FLAVOR PAIRING & WEIGHT LOSS COMBINATIONS — 52

4 QUICK START — 72

5 FREE BONUS: The Cinderella Accelerator And The Movement Sequencing Guide — 140

Readers are highly recommended to seek proper advice from either a physician or a professional practitioner before implementing any of these suggestions. Seriously, this book cannot replace professional and medical advice. Therefore, both the author and the publisher will not take any responsibility for any adverse results if readers really follow the information herein.

PART ONE: THE CINDERELLA SOLUTION EXPLAINED

1. THE CINDERELLA SOLUTION: "Weight Loss from the Inside-Out"

This IS the Last Time...

Before I explain the core premise of The Cinderella Solution (C.S.), I want you to consider how many times you have been here in the past. Whether you are in your 20's or 60's, one way or another, I know you must have tried to lose weight at some time in your life. While the motivation for embarking on a diet and/or exercise plan may have differed, the goal is generally the same for all of us – we want to look and feel better - The primary motivation is usually aesthetically driven.

"Secondary" incentives like overall health, energy, vitality and longevity typically take a back seat. This is human nature and we are all guilty - it's not a bad thing. However, it is actually those benefits perceived as secondary, that if healed correctly and set to optimal levels, will allow for rapid but more importantly permanent weight loss.

The main take-away here is that this isn't another 'quick-fix' that barks diet demands at you without telling you why you are doing what you are doing. Again, the goal here is to heal your body from the inside-out in order to feel what it's finally like to achieve fast, safe and permanent weight loss.

That means it's important to not only tell you how to do it but tell you why it works so well. In this book, The C.S. Main Book & Owner's Manual, I have done my best to be straight and to-the-point giving you all the information you need to get in the best shape of your life, while cutting out as much "fluff as possible".

I want you to get started as soon as possible but studies show that we are more likely to do something if we are told "why" we are doing it, along with the proof that it works.

WHERE & HOW TO GET STARTED

There are two ways to get started using the Cinderella Solution: The "Start NOW learn later" method or the "Learn NOW and start when I'm ready" method. Both work just as effectively, but we are all different and have different ways of getting things accomplished more effectively.

Cinderella Solution Your Complete System

Therefore, we have created this system so you can get started in whichever way you feel most comfortable:

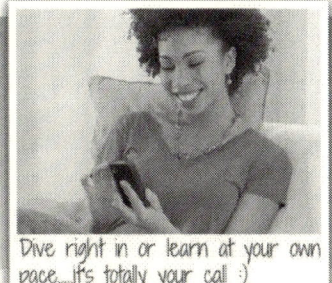

Dive right in or learn at your own pace....it's totally your call :)

TWO WAYS TO GET STARTED:

1. The "Start NOW learn later":

STEP 1). The C.S. Quick Start Guide
STEP 2). The C.S. Main Book & Owner's Manual

2. The "Learn NOW & start when I'm ready":

STEP 1). The C.S. Main Book & Owner's Manual
STEP 2). The C.S. Quick Start Guide

If you're ready to get rolling now, The C.S. Quick Start Guide will show you how to get started losing weight by tonight.

This is your daily manual that literally takes all the guess-work out of your journey by outlining all of your meals and what to do step-by-step in order to start your journey fast and finish your journey strong.

CINDERELLA SOLUTION

MAIN BOOK & OWNER'S MANUAL

Here you'll learn exactly how the flow of the system works as well as specific information on why it works so well.

You will learn about Cinderella's proven approach to weight loss rituals like "Flavor-Pairing" plus the two multi-faceted phases to get you there: 'Ignite and Launch'. Think of this as your detailed manual and reference guide to everything Cinderella :) After reading this book you'll have no questions on what to, when or how to do it.

2. WEIGHT LOSS RITUALS

Centuries old, proven-to-work rituals from the Planet's SLIMMEST, FITTEST AND HEALTHIEST Countries.

As you have already learned from my journey, after a while, the old-school methods like excess cardio, low carb diets and detoxes that most fitness and nutrition "guru's" advocate don't really work. Maybe if you're a guy or 22-years old with a lightning fast metabolism.... However, if you're reading this there's a

good chance that you don't fall into those categories.

The typical female metabolism is anything but typical and it takes more than the latest workout video to make a permanent change. The good news is that permanent change isn't rocket science, it just takes a little thinking outside the box....

THE PLANET'S HEALTHIEST COUNTRIES

It wasn't until my team and I started examining the world's healthiest nations that I knew we were on the right track. "Healthy" can mean a lot of different things to different people, however for most of us that means a leaner, more slender body. That operates at peak levels with the capacity to live a longer life.

This prompted us to dig deep into the practices of the world's healthiest countries to uncover what it was they were doing to stay more slender, feel better and live longer than we do in Westernized World. It turns out the differences were shocking!

The majority of our research proved that it wasn't so much about what they ate…instead it was more about how they ate. It's not that they exercised "more" - in fact these countries placed way less emphasis on the amount of exercise they did. The fittest nations all took a widely different approach to how they exercised in order to maintain their titles as "worlds healthiest countries."

It's not about WHAT you are doing – It's HOW you do it!

It all came down to the unique, usually unheard of "rituals" the people in these countries used to live longer, stay skinnier and feel better every single day. The good news was, as we dug even deeper, these countries didn't just become the world's healthiest nations….most of them had remained in the top-ten in multiple "worlds healthiest" rankers since researchers began rating them. This gave us the peace-of-mind knowing that not only did these rituals work, but they had been working for decades…. even centuries.

As you start your journey you'll have the same peace-of-mind knowing that the easy to follow and simple-to-start rituals like "Flavor-Pairing" & "Nutrient Timing" are the same tactics myself and thousands of other women have used to get our lives and our bodies back.

CINDERELLA'S CORE WEIGHT LOSS RITUAL CATEGORIES

The Cinderella Solution includes 4 Key Weight Loss Ritual Categories sourced from the fittest and healthiest countries in the world and are backed by the most up-to-date, unbiased research the scientific community has to offer.

In this section, we will dive into rituals that make Japan the skinniest country on the planet, habits that make Italians live longer than any other nation and an approach to exercise that makes the Netherlands #1 in fitness.

It's important to note that while we explain Cinderella's weight loss rituals in detail here, all of the "how's", "where's" and "when's" are taken care of for you and already implemented into your daily meal plans and recipes.

Here you will find out where our team was able to extract the rituals from, plus how and why they work. By digging into this section, you will not only be able to understand the foundation that makes Cinderella so effective, but you'll empower yourself with the knowledge needed to sustain these super- easy rituals after you've reset your metabolism and maintain your goal weight.

1. "FOOD-COUPLING"

"The ritual of combining the proper hormone influencing foods together for enhanced weight loss."

This ritual used heavily in Japan has allowed this country to load up on carbs for centuries while remaining in the world's skinniest county. This nation with the planets lowest Body Mass Index (BMI) takes in a whopping 55% of their daily food as Carbs!

This is even stranger considering that the world's highest BMI nation, The United States, doesn't even consume that percentage of daily carbs!

Their secret is not only what types of carbs, but how these carbs are coupled with other foods or "macronutrients". You see, in Japan starchy carbs like rice and potatoes are very rarely combined with high fat foods. Generally, you'll see these heavy carb meals coupled with a lean protein source like steak or fish.

By choosing high carb options that include a healthy dose of fiber, people in any country can "blunt" the insulin response that signals "fat storage". Along with this, both carbs and fiber create a "satiety-response" that tells your brain you are full so you avoid binge eating. Finally, Japan's top carb choices are gluten-free which have a positive effect on fat-loss hormones like cortisol and estrogen as well as digestion.

Food-Coupling Rules:

Try to couple higher carbohydrate meals with lean protein sources. Do not pair higher carb options with high fat options

Example: Skip traditional breakfasts like bacon, eggs & potatoes OR bagel & cream cheese, cereal & milk.

Try to choose carbohydrates that are rich in fiber to avoid fat storage

Example: Rice, potatoes, quinoa, oats etc.

Do not pair starchy carbs with sugar rich foods

Example: Most baked goods or even supposed "health foods" like trail-mix and granola (don't worry, we've got weight loss friendly recipes if you've got a sweet tooth)

Try to use gluten free carb options

Example: rice or rice-noodles, potatoes, gluten-free pasta.

2. "FLAVOR-PAIRING"

"The act of including specific seasonings and ingredients with meals to prompt a weight loss signal to your hormones."

The interesting thing about Flavor Pairing Rituals is that those who practice these habits rarely do it for its ability to keep them lean, healthy and energized. In most cases, specific seasonings, herbs, and natural sweeteners are specifically used to enhance taste. Many of these pairings have been proven to be the primary factors helping these countries rank among the skinniest nations in the world.

For example, some of the world's biggest consumers of spices like cinnamon and turmeric also happen to be ranked as #2 on the "world's lowest obesity list" at less than 5% (compared to >40% in the US). India is also listed as consistently having the lowest rate of degenerative diseases like Alzheimer's as well.

According to research we uncovered, there are certain foods or food flavorings that have the ability to not only signal your body to burn fat, but to energize, heal and prevent.

Continuing with the example of India's 2 favorite spices, spices like cinnamon have a positive effect on how well your insulin works which can prompt fat to be used as energy, rather than getting stored as fat on your hips and thighs.

Turmeric is a powerful spice that battles inflammation which is one of obesities direct causes. Antioxidants are inflammation's number one enemy and because of turmeric's extremely high antioxidant content, you can not only expect to reap weight loss benefits, but fight cancer, wrinkles and heart disease as well.

While Cinnamon and Turmeric are just two of Cinderella's flavor pairs, below we've listed the 3 more primary flavor pairings found in The Cinderella Solution. While you'll find more flavor, pairings infused into your day- to-day manual (Quick Start Guide), it's important to learn about how and why the simple act of adding specific seasonings can impact your ability to lose weight even more rapidly.

3 More Powerful Proven Flavor-Pairing Examples:

Cocoa/Chocolate: Proven to boost your weight-loss results by stimulating serotonin production in the brain while regulating your mood and helping suppress your appetite, which means you will consume less calories throughout the day.

+boost immune system +boost heart health +improve nails and hair +increase energy

Black Pepper: Like cinnamon and turmeric, black pepper blocks free radicals and has been proven reduce belly fat by blocking the formation of new fat cells. Studies show "piperine" (one of pepper's primary components) actually suppressed fat accumulation on a high sugar diet. Finally, pepper is also a thermogenic food – which causes the body to burn more calories at rest, as well as boosting the metabolism.

+natural anti-depressant +improved memory +improved digestion +increased estrogen elimination

Ginger: According to multiple studies ginger has the ability to produce many positive hormonal effects that signal weight loss, specifically with regards to insulin/blood sugar levels and leptin levels. In fact, in one study researchers concluded that ginger supplementation suppresses weight gain induced by a high fat diet and it might be a promising therapy for the treatment of obesity and its complications.

+REDUCE MUSCLE PAIN & SORENESS +LIMIT INFLAMATION +LOWER BLOOD SUGAR

3. "NUTRIENT-TIMING"

Knowing exactly when and how to "Food Couple" and "Flavor Pair" in order to create a more instant or prolonged weight loss effect.

In the past when you have tried to lose weight, you may have been eating the right foods, however you may not have been eating them at the right times. For example, Mediterranean countries like Italy, who are consistently ranked #1 on many of the world's slimmest and healthiest country lists, tend to eat a lot of high fat and protein sources, while skipping out on carbs for breakfast. This goes against the traditional North American breakfast that are carbohydrate rich (I'm sure you've even tried to eat healthy carb cereals yet still struggled with weight loss, right?).

Studies prove that by limiting carbs at breakfast and loading up on proteins and fats, you can actually promote an 18-hour fat burning effect. The science shows that a high fat/protein breakfast helps maintain optimal blood sugar levels from last night's dinner all the way until lunch the next day, prompting your body to burn fat for fuel for an extended time.

This is exactly how we have set up your meals and recipes during the first 14-day "Ignite" phase of eating in the Quick Start Guide While you'll load up on starchy carbs at lunch and fibrous carbs at dinner, we'll "do like the Roman's do" at breakfast by using a high fat/high protein meal to extend fat burning overnight and into the morning.

CARBS ARE <u>NOT</u> THE ENEMY!

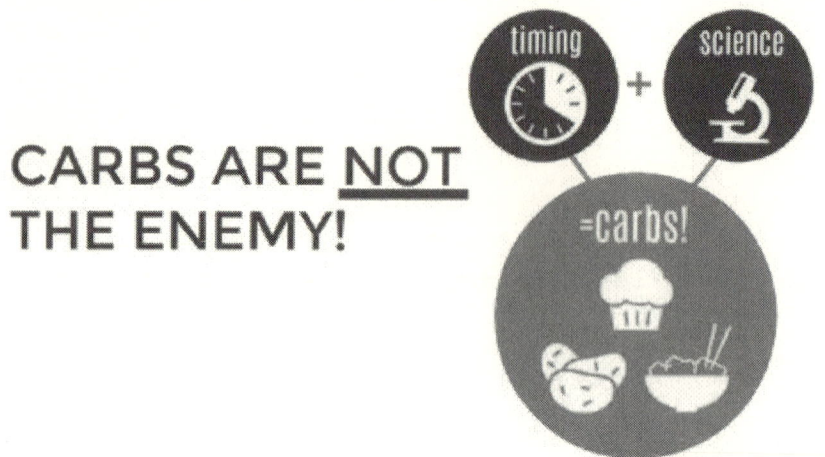

Don't worry you will still get to have your cherished carbs at breakfast in Cinderella's second phase, "Launch". You may be thinking, "what about my 18-hour fat-burning effect?" ...the problem is that the body "gets wise" to certain fat-loss principles, especially when you're losing weight as fast as you will within the first 2 weeks. As you will learn in the next chapter, we will add back the breakfast staples you are used to, and move the prolonged fat burning effect to later in the day.

Drink Wine and Still Lose Weight? YES PLEASE!!

The example of consuming a sugar-filled drink like wine, and still experiencing weight-loss, is the perfect example of proper Nutrient-Timing. Now, you have to make me a promise here....if I tell you the science of how to drink wine and still lose weight – you can't abuse it. This is one of those rare examples of "you CAN get too much of a good thing" so be responsible.

Ok here's the deal. Wine has a lot of sugar in it which can make your insulin/blood sugar/glucose levels rise. When you are trying to lose weight, this isn't good. When your glucose levels go up after consuming a meal high in sugary calories, there's a good chance those calories end up getting stored as fat. Also, not good. And when you think about it, usually when we drink wine we have during or close to a meal. Those additional sugar packed calories along with your meal (whether it be a healthy or not) signal your body to store most of those Cals as energy for later, otherwise known as a little extra fat on your belly and butt.

The trick here is that you must consume your wine 1.5 hours either before or after your last meal of the day. By timing the wine this way, one glass won't create an insulin surge that forces your body to store the entire meal as fatty tissue. Pretty cool right?

So, here's the quick tips on how to have a glass of wine here-and-there and still make the scale sing every time you step on it:

1) Nutrient-Time your wine 1.5 hours before or after your last meal

2.) Limit it to one glass per "wine-time".

3.) Remember the rule of calories in VS calories out still matters: If you're in the Launch Phase, skip your snack to make room for the wine. Or if you're in the Ignite Phase, do an extra "round" of one of the Movement-Sequencing Workouts to account for your wine Cals.

4)Stick to "dry" red wine as it has the least amount of calories.

And Finally, ...

While there are multiple ways to time the types of foods that go into your body the science is vast and could have a whole book dedicated to it – I know because our team has read them all. So, while we've outlined the importance of proper nutrition timing using the above example here, just remember that we have taken out all of the guess work for you in the Quick Start Guide.

4. "SLIM-SEQUENCING"

The proper exercise format, combined with unique exercises, that work with the female metabolism to enhance weight loss and muscle tone.

The foundation for The Cinderella Solution's exercise format really comes from looking at why North American exercise habits and methods have created the most obese continent on the planet. Unlike the world's fittest and leanest area, the Netherlands, we are an "all or nothing" culture. We either exercise our brains out or do nothing at all. It's either jump around like a maniac to a high-intensity workout DVD or binge watch a box set of Friends on DVD. Here it seems like we've evolved into a "Personal Trainer or Personal Pizza" nation.

The secret comes from countries like Denmark, Holland and Sweden who seem to have found a sort of "exercise balance". These countries simply exercise when they can and find ways to incorporate mini-workouts into their daily life. However, a big hurdle here was when we found out that these countries actually have set rules within the school and workplace that insist their students and employees exercise. Does your employer give you a lunch break or a workout break? In the Netherlands lunch breaks are called "Nutrition Breaks" and many employers give incentives like trips and money for staying fit.

With that in mind, we had to develop a way that allows for the same "exercise balance" enjoyed in the Netherlands. Our goal was to incorporate the most efficient and quick types of exercise into your already busy day. On top of that, you may not have time or may have no desire to go to the gym, so we've designed these workouts that you can do them in the comfort of your own living room.

That not only meant that the workouts had to be quick, but that they had to be as effective as possible in order to produce results as quickly as possible.

"Movement-Sequencing" does just that...

...by placing the right moves in the correct order, the female body has the ability to not only burn more calories during workout but burn more calories after the workout is complete as well. This is effective for rapid fat loss but helps work with one of your key fat-burning hormones Cortisol, as well.

Studies show exercising for long periods of time cause havoc in your adrenal glands, spiking cortisol and prompting deadly visceral fat to land on your belly and around your organs. This is why we've ensured that your workouts can be done in 6-22 minutes in order to get the most out of your limited time to exercise.

And finally, speaking of "stress", we don't want you stressing about exercising every day or only for 6 minutes if that's all you have time for. The nutrition rituals and done-for-you meal plans in your Quick Start Guide are so effective that using the "Movement Sequencing Guide" in your Accelerator Package is not compulsory. Yes, it's true that incorporating exercise as you feel comfortable WILL enhance the speed of your transformation, but please let the food do the work. When you're ready to increase the amount of weight you're losing, then you'll find a way to increase the exercise component.

AND REMEMBER,

For an extremely detailed guide that outlines even more of the Flavor

Pairing Rituals and Weight Loss Combinations, refer to the final part (4) in this book "Flavor Pairing and Weight Loss Combinations" on page 82. Here you'll find the Top 10 fat burning habits and how to incorporate them into your daily routine.

If you are looking for more insight on Food-Coupling techniques and how to build your own meals using these principles, you can skip ahead to Part 3, "DIY Meal Creator & Flavor Pairing" on Page 60.

Keep in mind if you're looking to get started and take any additional "brain work" out of the equation, Check out the pre-designed meals and recipes in your Quick Start Guide.

3. IGNITE & LAUNCH: "Cinderella's 2-Phase Approach to weight loss"

"AND WE'RE OFF!"

If you've ever been to the track or watched a horse race on TV, sometimes you see a horse that looks as though it gets shot out of the gate and flies around the track. It effortlessly leaves every other horse miles behind, only to cross the finish line looking like he was ready to take another lap. This is the equivalent of Cinderella's second phase, 'Launch'.

However, the owners of that horse didn't just line him up at the starting gate and hope for the best. Built into that horse is the best training that money could buy, the best food and supplementation governed by a superior jockey on top. There's a good chance that the owners and trainers employed a lot of techniques and tactics that its competitors either missed, or simply did not do. A lot of work happened behind the scenes to engineer such a superior animal and

Cinderella Solution Your Complete System

guarantee a winner. This is the equivalent to Cinderella's first phase, 'Ignite'.

PLEASE NOTE:

In the following sections, you will learn about *how* and *why* the Ignite and Launch phases are used in the Cinderella Solution. While all the tactics, principles and explanations behind these approaches are explained in detail, just remember that everything is always laid out for you in an easy-to-follow format in the Quick Start Guide. All the guess work is taken care of, however the following sections will allow you to truly master Cinderella Solution's daily operations.

PHASE 1: THE IGNITE PHASE (14 DAYS)

The Ignite Phase is the preparation and engineering that will not only make this your most successful attempt ever at getting in shape, but will ensure that it's the last time you ever have to do it, as well. Ignite's measures are all the key actions taken leading up to the successful race (Launch, the second 14-day phase). Here in Ignite, we will reset hormones and heal the organs that deliver those hormones to ensure rapid fat loss. While we've taken a lot of time to create recipes and meal combinations, this will still be the toughest of the two phases.

Exercise, foods and their pairings are reviewed here. They are tactically designed to reverse insulin-resistance, cortisol-abundance and enhance estrogen regulation for longevity, weight loss and overall health.

1.) Reset Insulin management systems

2.) Reduce Cortisol levels

3.) Regulate Estrogen levels.

Not only will this significantly enhance your capacity to burn fat and manage food more efficiently, but we've engineered this phase to improve mental well-being, detoxify your liver and kidneys while enhancing the digestive process.

There are a lot of positive internal changes that may come with some "uncomfortable" feelings when you do this phase on your first run through. However, just like anything else that results in a massively positive outcome, just "take comfort in any discomfort". And don't worry, all I'm talking about is the occasional headache and maybe some irritability in the first few days of Ignite. Weight loss will come fast here because not only are your hormones being set to optimal levels which is highly conducive for weight loss, but we are ultimately leaving your body no other option but to use your fat as fuel.

IGNITE GOALS & TARGETS:

- Regulate foods that cause insulin sensitivity and resistance so that your body manages sugar more efficiently, thus making it extremely difficult for your body to store any food as fat on your body.
- Eliminate and/or moderate substances that increase cortisol and stress levels in order to heal adrenal glands, thus promoting fat elimination on your stomach as well as, in and around your organs.
- Introduce foods, flavor pairings and food combinations that up- regulate or downgrade estrogen levels to optimal, as well as enhance estrogen elimination. While you will see positive changes in mood, digestion and energy, you will also witness fat reduction specifically in the hips, butt and thighs.
- Maintain a three meal per day schedule to alleviate digestive stress, enhance estrogen elimination and promote nutrient uptake
- Introduce herbs, spices and dressings that help the liver and kidneys' detoxification process to help break down fat to use as energy.
- Use workouts and exercise (if you're ready to) that are designed to get the entire body used to working as a complete unit and promote natural growth hormone production allowing increases in fat incineration.
- Enlist "anaerobic" exercise principles rather than traditional aerobic training (cardio specific) to maintain optimal cortisol levels and enhance insulin/glycogen management.

PHASE 2: THE LAUNCH PHASE (14 DAYS)

Welcome to everyone's favorite phase, the Cinderella "Launch" Phase. We'll be adding foods like grains, fruit and even more carb-rich recipes! These will significantly enhance your metabolic fires AND make meals ultra-tasty. This is the part in the race where you seem to 'launch' out of the gate and glide past everyone else. Traditional diets often have you losing about a pound of muscle for every pound of fat you lose, leaving your body soft and begging to gain all the weight back. Here in Launch, we'll do the exact opposite.

Exercise, foods and their pairings are reviewed here. They are tactically designed to continue improving on enhanced insulin, cortisol and estrogen maintenance "primed" during the Ignite phase

1.) Optimize Thyroid Production

2.) Reduce Inflammation and Acidity

3.) Increase Fat-Burning Hormones, Testosterone and Human Growth Hormone

4.) Set Your Hunger-Hormone Leptin to Optimal Levels for Fat-Burning

As a result of the extra energy that you will be able to bring to your optional workouts, you will be burning amplified amounts of fat hours after they are complete. In turn, you will forge new, feminine muscle increasing the percentage of the fat you burn on a daily basis. It gets better. Along with that, fat-burning hormones like testosterone and growth hormone will be turned up as well. Finally, here you will see specific victories with regards to decreased dress sizes, inches lost (as the focus will be on changes in your body's composition) and how "toned" you look.

LAUNCH GOALS & TARGETS

- Re-introduce foods absent from Ignite that will now be utilized more efficiently following hormone regulation.
- Introduce new and increased amounts of 'Power Carbs', plus food combinations that provide sustainable energy to workout with more intensity providing enhanced, all-day, fat-burning effects.

- Optimize your hormone Leptin, a hormone produced in your fat cells, to increase fat burning and prevent hunger.
- Increase exercise induced fat-burning by increasing intensity and specialization within workouts to build lean tissue that significantly enhances metabolic speed and proficiency.
- Increase the efficiency of the endocrine system (primarily the thyroid gland) to optimize production, storage and the release of hormones into the bloodstream which consequently increases the efficiency in the delivery to cells.
- Add and diversify 'Prime Protein' sources in order to forge and maintain levels of feminine muscle, plus increase cell repair within the muscle.
- Increase the amount of meals per day to four while decreasing portion sizes to increase available energy, stabilize blood sugar and significantly enhance your metabolism.

If you are adding the right types of carbs at the right times like you will in the Launch Phase, you don't have to worry about gaining weight – as you'll see, the opposite is true!

CYCLING THE IGNITE & LAUNCH PHASES

- Your first phase Ignite, lasts a total of 14 days followed by the Launch phase which also lasts 14 days. As mentioned before, always begin with the Ignite phase and then move to the Launch phase.
- If you have not reached your goal weight following completion of the IGNITE & LAUNCH phases (first 28days), you will then 'RE-IGNITE' and move back to the IGNITE phase again for another 14 days/2 weeks. After this second IGNITE phase, you will "RE-LAUNCH" and move to the LAUNCH phase again for another 14 days/2 weeks.

You will follow this protocol of switching back and forth between Ignite and launch every 14 days until you reach your goal.

4. CINDERELLA MACROS & FOOD PAIRING RITUALS

MACRONUTRIENTS EXPLAINED

There are three major macronutrients your body needs in order to function properly including carbohydrates, protein and fats. While these three major macronutrient groups can include many sources of food, by now you know that not all foods are created equal.

In creating The Cinderella Solution, we designed a rigorous criteria for selection and inclusion of specific foods. Although we are concerned with what's in these foods, we have also taken the added step to evaluate what happens hormonally and metabolically when you digest these foods.

- Protein is one of the three key macronutrients that make up the food we eat. While the macronutrient ratios of all the protein sources we eat (fish, pork, eggs, etc.) can vary, each gram of protein contains 4 calories. Our primary focus in
- C.S. is not calories but more importantly, the 'quality' of the calories provided from the protein source.
- With reference to quality, "C.S. Prime Proteins" are proteins selected based on multiple factors however, the two big ones are: 1.) "Bio-Availability" which is your body's ability to absorb the nutrients and make available for use by your body and 2) Genetic makeup which relies on a number of factors including macronutrient ratios and the general practices used to raise that particular protein (e.g. Grain-fed beef VS factory-farmed beef).

- When selecting protein sources, please do your best to look for those labeled 'Responsibly Raised', organic, grass fed/finished, wild caught, free range etc. While this is not imperative, results may be significantly enhanced by taking the time to select animal proteins that adhere to more responsible farming practices.

Eating the RIGHT kinds of protein burns more calories than any other macronutrient.

PRIME PROTIENS
IGNITE & LAUNCH SPECIFIC GUIDELINES

✓ It is definitely more important to reach for more 'responsibly raised' proteins during the Ignite Phase, as we are trying to reset hormones to optimal levels. This will help cleanse your body of unhealthy bacteria, additional estrogen as well as 'superbugs' that can inhibit this goal.

Again, this is not imperative, as it can be tough to find. If you can't find more "responsibly raised" animal proteins, the good news is that this plan provides a strong detox-factor which will help with elimination of bacteria and hormones.

✓ While lean sources of <u>beef and pork are exempt during the Ignite Phase</u>, they are included during Launch. This is because we are trying to improve digestion and prime the metabolism during Ignite, and these particular protein sources are more difficult to digest. Once this task is completed, we will add them back in the Launch phase and utilize them for their thermogenic/anabolic (fat burning, muscle sparing or building) properties.

o Fat is another one of the three major macronutrients and contains 9 calories per gram which is more than double the calories found in protein and carbs. Even though its caloric content is higher, it is a mistake to avoid it (as is adopted by many other nutrition systems).

o What we do need to do here, is be cautious of the quality and the type of fat that you include with your meals.

o The absolute best fat sources, "Royal Fats", can actually help amplify fat-loss and reset hormones for continued success. Therefore, we have selected naturally occurring fat sources comprised of Omega 3 and 6 fatty acids, monounsaturated, polyunsaturated and some saturated fat in healthy amounts. The key here is to avoid man-made fats that find their way into 40% of the products on supermarket shelves such as trans-fats.

ROYAL FATS
IGNITE AND LAUNCH SPECIFIC GUIDELINES

- ✓ In terms of sources, Royal Fats remain the same throughout both phases coming from nuts and seeds, dairy-free milks and butters, as well as other sources like avocados and olives.

- ✓ In the Ignite Phase you will be eating more fat in any given meal which will encourage your body to use your stored fat as fuel. However, to maintain the effectiveness of this tactic, we will taper down the fats during the Launch phase and increase carbohydrate consumption.

This will not only keep metabolic fires burning, but provide an energy source with increased efficiency for your more demanding workouts in the Launch phase.

o Just like fats and proteins, all carbohydrates are not created equal however, all carbohydrates have 4 calories per gram.

- Specific classes of carbs are used, metabolized and digested differently which is why we have separated them into two distinct categories, 'Power Carbs' and 'Angel Carbs'. While most traditional diets and nutrition systems over the last three decades aim to eliminate carbohydrates, this mistake is one of the major contributors to the "yo-yo" diet epidemic, as well as the culprit for many plateaus that you've encountered on these plans.

- In C.S., the biggest bonus of 'power carbs' is that they are 'starchy' in nature and provide a superior energy source without an immediate spike in insulin.

- As we've mentioned before, everything you do throughout C.S. will be done tactically and with both precision and purpose therefore, we'll be doing the same with your carbs. Gone are the carbs that significantly impede digestion, cause allergenic responses (gluten) and cause dramatic spikes (added sugars) in insulin.

POWER CARBS
IGNITE & LAUNCH SPECIFIC GUIDELINES

- During the Launch phase, you will increase your Power Carb intake as you'll need more usable energy to get through your workouts. Although the workouts are not long, the intensity you bring to your workouts in Launch is the key. These extra carbs will provide the extra sustainable energy boost you need.

- Gluten-free grains and fruits are added during the Launch phase while they are absent from the first phase, Ignite. It's not that these foods are "bad" for you, however they are omitted in Ignite because we are making an all-out attempt to reset hormones. And for some, these items can provide less than optimal digestive, cortisol and insulin related responses. After achieving hormonal and digestive balance in phase one (Ignite) the positive effects of fruits and grains will be more effective upon reintroduction.

PLEASE NOTE: Some of us simply don't do well with grains, even if they are gluten-free. Depending upon your individual digestive system (as well as cultural background) you may have some sort of "hitch" when it comes to grains, ranging from minor issues, to an intolerance to gluten-free grains. The good news is, even if a tolerance problem has not been identified, you'll know upon reintroduction in the Launch phase. Although unlikely, (roughly 5-10% of the population) you could experience digestive issues such as bloating and irregularities. If this happens upon starting the Launch phase and is persistent over a few days, it may be a good idea to substitute grains with the other Power Carbs listed. Don't worry buddy, you don't have to remove them for your life forever, just get through this without them for now and pick your battles later on. Again, this is highly unlikely but ultimately, I just want to ensure your success and make sure all our bases are covered.

ANGEL CARBS

- o Just like all carbohydrates, there are 4 calories per gram in 'Angel Carbs'. These carbs differ from 'Power Carbs' because of their limited starch content and the fact that Angel Carbs are always vegetable based.
- o While there are multiple varieties of vegetables, "angel carbs" have been specifically selected for their "angelic qualities" that help with hormone optimization and overall health, vitality and longevity. Our guidelines for the selection of "Angel Carbs" includes many cruciferous vegetables, vitamin c content, fiber content and many more.
- o Angel carbs are also characterized by their ability to reduce insulin spikes and help with the management and delivery of nutrients from other foods.

ANGEL CARBS
IGNITE AND LAUNCH SPECIFIC GUIDELINES

- ✓ Throughout both Ignite and Launch, your selection of Angel Carbs remains the same.

- ✓ Portion sizes listed in your Ignite and Launch "Daily Meal Guides" are set minimum requirements for "Angel Carbs". All this means is that when it comes to vegetables, the portion sizes listed are a minimum and you may have as much as you like. However, remember to stick to the portion sizes listed for Prime Proteins, Royal Fats and Power Carbs. While we don't want you going overboard here, we also never want to hear that you're always hungry either.

- ✓ If you are hungry between meals (which I doubt you will be), you may have 1-2 cups of any Angel Carbs. Use this advice if you are between meals and absolutely need some food or energy. Remember though, some hunger about an hour prior to eating a meal is alright (and normal) and a great indicator that your metabolism and digestion is gaining speed!

And Just Remember...

As you'll see in the Quick Start Guide that you will be following, this is another component that is totally done for you with all of the guess work taken out. However, as we've mentioned before, we feel it is always important tell you "why" you are doing what you're doing and understand the premise. Embracing the tactical reasoning behind all these principles will not only increase your chances of success, but ensure you maintain it as well!!!

5. MEAL TIMING & FREQUENCY

'LOSS LEADERS' AND 'GURU WARS'

The concept of when to eat your meals and how many to eat is up for debate between self-proclaimed You Tube gurus, legitimate registered dietitians and everyone in between. With all the different opinions (usually conflicted), it can be tough to figure out what to do. More importantly, what's best for you. Some say 6 to 8 mini-meals is the answer, some say 1 or 2, and some will even tell you to fast all day and gorge the next. Who or what is right?

For your peace of mind, I will answer this question based on what has been a victory for the thousands of clients that have successfully graduated from my programs. I will also provide you with up-to-date scientific facts on why it is going to work for you. The bottom line, and the most important part, is in fact that calories do count. You already know, that if you eat more than your body needs for too long, you are most likely going to gain weight, and more specifically, gain fat. Alternatively, if you eat too little for too long you are likely going to stop losing weight and plateau.

The Cinderella Solution emphasizes the idea of "tactical precision" throughout. This includes the type of calories consumed and how it effects your body. All of your efforts could be for nothing if the number of calories (or energy) you consume, is more or less than you need.

I know you might be wondering, "So, what do I do?".

Don't worry, it's all been taken care of for you...

'What' and "how much" you are going to eat is outlined in the, Daily Meal Guides.So that's all squared away for you with no guess work. Plus, we have also designed this system in order to allow you pick your own meals and foods while still managing the perfect calorie and macronutrient counts

All you have to do is figure out 'when' you are going to eat your meals. It's super simple, and here's the plan on the following page:

IGNITE PHASE: 3 MEALS DAILY

The reason for 3 separate meals is both scientific and strategic. While many experts will have you eating 5 to 6 mini-meals a day, boasting that it will speed your metabolism, that theory is flawed.

Your metabolism is relative to what you eat, how much you eat, your hormonal balance and digestion. With a hormonal storm raging inside, you will invoke a hormonal traffic jam inside that eating 10 of the tiniest meals daily couldn't fix. Relative to that analogy, this is what could also cause a 10-car pileup in your intestines if you are not processing food efficiently and eliminating what you don't need with speed.

That's why in Ignite we focus hard on hormonal optimization and digestion. It's the standard issue BLD - Breakfast, Lunch and Dinner. You'll eat three meals per day using the most perfect foods for optimization. Limiting your meals to three each day will allow for the ideal time for digestion, delivery and assimilation of healing nutrients and start the elimination process. Let's face it, finding time to prep and eat 5 - 6 meals a day can be overwhelming and totally unrealistic, Right?

LAUNCH PHASE: 4 MEALS DAILY

In the Launch Phase we are going to sneak in one extra meal. Remember in Launch, we bump up your carb-count a little, so rather than squeeze in more than you need at any given meal and impede digestion, you will add a fourth meal.

By now we have optimized digestion during the Ignite phase, so your body can handle that additional meal. Also, with enhanced metabolism, digestion, delivery and elimination you could be hungrier more often - that fourth meal will take care of that. Finally, to make things easier, the fourth additional meal will usually look more like a snack that is easy to make and quick to consume.

Just to be clear, there is no compelling evidence that suggests eating smaller meals more frequently leads to additional weight loss. Our reasoning for adding the fourth meal is because we have optimized your hormone levels and digestion (throughout Ignite) therefore you could be hungrier in Launch. The big take away here, is that with hunger comes cravings, and with cravings comes....well you know. Our ultimate goal is to keep you on track. That extra meal ensures continuous weight loss and prevents overindulgences that could throw you off track biologically and mentally.

WHEN TO EAT

When you wake up

In terms of when to eat these meals, it's up to you, kind of. You're a busy lady so just be sure to get Breakfast/Meal 1 within two hours of waking up. Some 'experts' will say that eating immediately will "wake up your metabolism" which is an arbitrary phrase and isn't always true. Some say that waiting as long as possible will allow you to burn more fat for longer, which is true to a certain extent, but can be detrimental as well.

Your best option is to eat whenever it is convenient, within those first two hours. Don't you dare miss this meal though, even if you are not hungry. You can also eat about 30 minutes to an hour before you exercise in the morning or, directly after. By doing this you can achieve all the benefits of eating as soon as you wake up (waking up the metabolism theory) or, wait a while to eat (extending the caloric burn from sleep). The choice here is yours based on routine or convenience and will no doubt keep your body guessing, as well as aid in plateau prevention.

During the Day:

As for the meals that follow Breakfast/Meal 1, you will try to separate them by 3 to 4 hours until you reach your final meal of the day. This will allow significant time for digestion, assimilation and delivery of things like vitamins and minerals. While most people are not hungry between meals, some may feel as though they're starving. Regardless, experiencing some hunger is a good sign. For some, this may be an indicator that their metabolic processes are speeding up, while for others it could indicate that you were eating too much prior to becoming a future Cinderella Success Story. What we are truly aiming for is some hunger prior to the next meal.

A herbal tea between meals not only kills cravings but many have properties that fight fat as well!

SPECIAL NOTE: If you feel as though you are extremely hungry between meals, reach for a serving of 'Angel Carbs' that will fill you up without disrupting insulin levels (which we are looking to optimize). You also have the option to have an herbal tea here as well. You may be thinking, "but I'm hungry, what's a tea going to do?". The answer is, "Usually a lot." because sometimes we experience a sort of "pseudo hunger". Remember, this system is set up so you're consistently getting enough food so, sometimes your brain could be sending you mixed messages. This could be from thirst, or simply a craving brought on by something you see on TV or even photo of something delicious on-line. A pomegranate tea with stevia can satisfy a sugar craving, while a minty cocoa tea will satisfy your need for chocolate.

For Dinner:

Finally, do your best to make sure that you eat your last meal about 2 - 3 hours before going to bed. This is another subject up for debate, but again we'll turn to the results of the thousands of our most successful clients, as well as some hard evidence to settle the matter.

From the jump, I've always asked clients to make sure they "close the kitchen" by about 7 pm. Some people listen better than others, but when comparing clients' food journals, it's always the ones that listen to these little tricks that lose the most weight, the fastest. This fact is driven home by research studies that show the same conclusions as well. In a group of 29 people, participants lost an extra pound over the 2 weeks in the study when they eliminated food between 7pm and 6am. When given 2 more weeks on the same diet and asked to eat later than 7pm, they gained weight – over a pound. There are many factors that influence weight loss with night time fasting, but just consider that although the body is a complex machine, it can only do so much at once. If it's focusing on digestion, it's not as focused on burning fat or even getting a deep sleep which is of greater importance. Deep sleep is related not only to balancing the ICE hormones but increasing fat burning hormones like testosterone and IGF-1.

PART TWO: MEAL CREATEOR & FLAVOR PAIRING

Until now you've been told by the media and the self-proclaimed gurus to go low-carb, low-fun, watch-the-fat, take-this-pill - so I can completely understand why you're wondering how these simple habits can lead to such dramatic results. The truth is other quick-fix solutions and fad approaches work for some people but for most of us, especially women, we need an approach that works with our bodies to promote change from the inside-out.

In our time of need (or when we're desperate) we latch on to ideas that sound good in theory, but in reality, only work for some. Low-Fat diets, Ketogenic plans and many other popular diets essentially force weight loss from the outside in – essentially its blunt force trauma that scares your body into saying, "I better lose weight or else". But the truth is, as soon as you deviate from the plan your body is relieved and wants to find its old equilibrium – or go back to the way it was before you tried these shock tactics.

This is what myself, along with many scientists and doctors I met with, blame the yo-yo diet epidemic on. What's worse is that these methods actually "break" your Metabolism forcing you to gain more weight that you had before, while making it harder to lose weight when trying the next fad approach....

No More!

It's time to "promote change from the inside out". Whether you choose to use this DIY approach or use the pre-made meals we have provided, over the next few weeks you will see, and almost more importantly, FEEL what it's like when your body is gently pushed in the right direction, rather than beaten into submission.

Essentially proper food-combinations and timing is like hitting the "Fat- Flush" button on your three major fat loss hormones -Insulin, Cortisol and Estrogen. Instead of deprivation or taking away a vital element needed for your body's day-today operations (fat-free, low-carb, starvation diets), you will be creating the perfect hormonal environment needed for your body to release the fat that it's been holding onto over the last few years.

That's why instead of feeling tired, hungry and depressed like you do on these other plans, this time you'll actually feel energized and happy, along with a big sense of renewal. And don't forget, of course you'll be rewarded on the scale, as well as how you look in the mirror too.

3 STEP INSTRUCTION GUIDE

LETS GET STARTED - EASY AS 1, 2, 3

STEP #1

REVIEW YOUR "IGNITE"(first 2 week phase) & LAUNCH (second 2 week phase) FOOD PAIRING LEGENDS

- We know you are busy, so we've done our best to streamline everything to take any extra steps out of the equation. Keeping this in mind, we have broken up the method on how you choose to portion your food into two separate categories: "Free Hand" & "The Weigh-Way.
- The Free Hand Method detailed on Page 73 simply allows you to use your hand and as guide for portioning your food i.e.: 1 Palm of turkey breast, 1 thumb almond butter etc.
- The "Weigh-Way" is just like it sounds and is the more traditional, more time- consuming method of weighing your food. Although it can take a little bit more time, this method might be better if you have the time or prefer a little more order in your life.
- As you will see in you Food-Blocks section (page 75) each of these methods are listed beside the food lists for Prime Proteins, Royal Fats, Power Carbs and Angel Carbs.

STEP #2

Choose a portion system that you wish to follow the Food Blocks on part there

- Your Transformation will be broken down into 2 separate phases : "Ignite" &
- "Launch"
- For the first 2 weeks you will follow the Ignite Phase, directly followed by the Launch Phase for another 4 weeks
- Your Food Pairing Legend for weeks 1 and 2 (Ignite) is located.
- Your Food Pairing Legend for weeks 3-4 Launch is located.
- On these pages you will see a chart listing your meals for the day with corresponding numbers in the Prime Protein, Royal Fats, Power Carbs and Angel Carb categories.
- The numbers listed beside the meal represent your "Food Blocks". These are
- the set portions for that specific meal.
- All of your "Food Blocks" represent a specific portion, or amount of food that you will eat at each meal. You will find your "Food Blocks" for Prime Proteins, Royal Fats, Power Carbs & Angel Carbs.

More on all this in a second, it'll all come together by the end of step 3 :)

STEP #3

Put it all together and create your Meals

- This is the part that makes this system super easy and even more effective: When choosing your meals for a given day, all you have to do is select your favorite foods from the Food-Blocks Section
- **For example,**
    - if your Food-Pairing Legend asks you to have 1 "Block" of Prime Protein, you could choose to have 2oz, or a ½ palm of Turkey Breast.
    - If it asks you to have 2 Blocks of Royal Fats, you could have 2 tsp's, or 2 forefingers of olive oil. Here, because it asks you for 2 Blocks in your Meal Legend you would multiply the portion listed in the Food Blocks section by 2. (2 blocks of Royal Fats X 1 tsp. olive oil = 2tsp olive oil.
    - If it asks you to have a 1 Block of Power Carbs, you could choose to have a 1/2 cup, or 1 palm of cooked quinoa.
    - And finally, Angel Carbs are always unlimited, so you may choose to have whatever choice, in whatever amount as a base for your meal.
    - Once it's all put together you'll have a delicious, fat burning Turkey & Quinoa Medley on a bed of fresh greens.

IGNITE & LAUNCH MEAL LEGENDS

food-pairing meal legends

These are the Food-Pairing Legends you will use during the Ignite and Launch Phases to create your meals. The corresponding food blocks/portions with food choices for Prime Proteins, Royal Fats, Power Carbs and Angel Carbs are found starting on page 75.

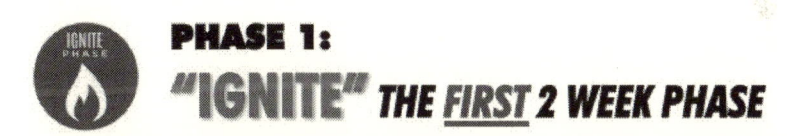

PHASE 1:
"IGNITE" THE FIRST 2 WEEK PHASE

IGNITE MEAL	PRIME PROTEIN	ROYAL FAT	POWER CARB	ANGEL CARB
BREAKFAST	2	2	0	UNLIMITED
LUNCH	2	1	2	UNLIMITED
DINNER	2	2	0	UNLIMITED

PHASE 2:
"LAUNCH" *THE SECOND 2 WEEK PHASE*

LAUNCH MEAL	PRIME PROTEIN	ROYAL FAT	POWER CARB	ANGEL CARB
BREAKFAST	1	1	1	UNLIMITED
LUNCH	1	2	0	UNLIMITED
SNACK*	1 OR 1		+ 1	UNLIMITED/OPTIONAL
DINNER	2	1	0	UNLIMITED

PORTIONING OPTIONS

measuring your food: portion options

Below are the 2 methods you can use to portion out your food for any given meal. While the "Free Hand Method" offers you a quick and easy way to build your meals by using portions of your hand to measure food, "The Weigh-Way" gives you a little more control if you feel you need it. Depending on your lifestyle and the amount of control you desire, both methods, or a combination of the two will do the trick!

FOOD & PORTION BLOCKS

In your IGNITE BREAKFAST Food Legend, you are asked to have:

2 PRIME PROTEINS, 2 ROYAL FATS, 0 POWER CARBS & UNLIMITED ANGEL CARBS.

FOR EXAMPLE

MEAL	PRIME PROTEIN	ROYAL FAT	POWER CARB	ANGEL CARB
BREAKFAST	2	2	0	UNLIMITED

PRIME PROTEIN	ROYAL FAT	POWER CARB	ANGEL CARB
2 =	2 =	0 =	UNLIMITED
2/3 C. EGG WHITES	1 WHOLE EGG + 1 TBSP OLIVE OIL	N/A	MUSHROOMS & RED PEPPER

Say you would like to make an omelette for breakfast, all you have to do is simply refer to the Food Block/Portion pages that follow and build your meal. Portion sizes for "Free Hand" measurement and "The Weigh Way" are both listed to make everything super quick and really easy.

Prime PROTEINS

BEST

FOOD CHOICE	QUICK MEASURE	EXACT MEASUREMENT
SARDINES	1/2 PALM	2 OZ. (2 MEDIUM SIZED)
BONELESS SKINLESS CHICKEN	1 PALM+	2 OZ. COOKED / 3 OZ RAW
EGG WHITES	N/A	3 LARGE OR 1/3 CUP
ANCHOVIES	1 PALM	3 OZ.
PROTEIN POWDER	N/A	1 TBSP (ROUNDED)
WHITE FISH (COD, TILAPIA ETC)	1 PALM+	3 OZ. COOKED / 4 OZ. RAW
SALMON/TUNA	1 PALM	2 OZ. COOKED / 3 OZ. RAW
GAME MEAT	1 PALM	2 OZ. COOKED / 3 OZ. RAW
GROUND TURKEY OR CHICKEN	1 PALM	2 OZ. COOKED / 3 OZ. RAW
RED MEAT (EXTRA LEAN)	1 PALM	2 OZ. COOKED / 3 OZ. RAW

BETTER

FOOD CHOICE	QUICK MEASURE	EXACT MEASUREMENT
LOX, SALMON	½ PALM	2OZ. RAW
ALMOND MILK	N/A	1 CUP
TURKEY BACON	N/A	2 SLICES
PORK TENDERLOIN	1 PALM	2OZ. COOKED / 3OZ RAW
SKINLESS CHICKEN THIGH/DRUM	1 PALM	2OZ COOKED / 3 OZ. RAW
TURKEY/HAM SLICES, DELI	1 PALM	3 OZ./2 SLICES
TURKEY BREAKFAST SAUSAGE	N/A	1 SAUSAGE
GROUND BEEF, EXTRA LEAN	1 PALM	2 OZ. COOKED/ 3 OZ. RAW
CLAMS/MUSSELS/SHRIMP	1 FIST	4 OZ. COOKED/ 6 OZ RAW

GOOD

VEGAN & VEGETARIAN (and super-picky eater) **OPTIONS**

While the animal-friendly options below are healthy, foods that contain dairy and soy in larger amounts can impede hormonal function and thus, weight loss. Feel free to use these options, but be sure to use them sparingly.

FOOD CHOICE	QUICK MEASURE	EXACT MEASUREMENT
GREEK YOGURT	3/4 FIST	3/4 CUP
COTTAGE CHEESE	1 PALM	1/2 CUP
VEGGIE BURGER	N/A	1 SMALL PATTY (3 OZ.)
TEMPEH	1 PALM	2 OZ.
TOFU, EXTRA FIRM	1 PALM	3 OZ.
VEGGGIE-BACON	N/A	2 SLICES (1 OZ.)

Royal FATS

	FOOD CHOICE	QUICK MEASURE	EXACT MEASUREMENT
BEST	AVACADO	2 THUMBS	1/4 SMALL-MEDIUM AVOCADO
	ALMONDS	1 THUMB	1 TBSP. CHOPPED/6 WHOLE
	CASHEWS	1 THUMB	1 TBSP. CHOPPED/4 WHOLE
	PUMPKIN SEEDS	1 THUMB+	2 TBSP.
	PECANS	1 THUMB	1 TBSP. CHOPPED/5 HALVES
	CHIA SEEDS	1 THUMB	2 ½ TSP.
	PISTACIOS	1 THUMB	1 TBSP. CHOPPED/10 WHOLE
	FLAX SEEDS, GROUND	1 THUMB	1 TBSP.
	SUNFLOWER SEEDS	1 THUMB	1 TBSP.
	SESAME SEEDS	1 THUMB	1 TBSP.
BETTER	EXTRA-VIRGIN OLIVE OIL	1 FOREFINGER TIP	1 TSP
	CHIA OIL	1 FOREFINGER TIP	1 TSP
	1 WHOLE EGG	N/A	1 SMALL
	ALMOND BUTTER	1 FOREFINGER TIP	1 ½ TSP.
	CASHEW BUTTER	1 FOREFINGER TIP	1 ½ TSP.
	PUMPKIN SEED OIL	1 FOREFINGER TIP	1 TSP
	COCONUT OIL/BUTTER	1 FOREFINGER TIP	1 TSP
	SHREDDED COCONUT, UNSWEET	2 THUMBS	2 TBSP
	COCONUT MILK, CANNED	2 THUMBS	5 TSP

VEGAN & VEGETARIAN (and super-picky eaters) **OPTIONS**

While the animal-friendly options below are healthy, foods that contain dairy and soy in larger amounts can impede hormonal function and thus, weight loss. Feel free to use these options, but be sure to use them sparingly.

	FOOD CHOICE	QUICK MEASURE	EXACT MEASUREMENT
GOOD	FETA CHEESE	2 THUMBS	2 LEVEL TBSP.
	GOAT CHEESE	2 THUMBS	2 LEVEL TBSP.
	REAL MOZZARELLA	1 THUMB	2 LEVEL TBSP
	PARMESAN CHEESE (low sodium)	2 THUMBS	2 LEVEL TBSP. GRATED

Power CARBS

	FOOD CHOICE	QUICK MEASURE	EXACT MEASUREMENT
BEST	QUINOA	1 PALM	1/3 CUP COOKED
	WHITE OR BROWN RICE	1 PALM	1/3 CUP COOKED
	WILD RICE	1 PALM	1/3 CUP COOKED
	BEETS	N/A	2 MEDIUM
	PARSNIP	1 FIST MASHED	1 MEDIUM SIZE
	SWEET POTATO	1 FIST MASHED	1/2 MEDIUM SIZE
	SQUASH	2 FISTS	2 CUPS CUBED
	APPLES	N/A	1 SMALL
	PEARS	N/A	1 SMALL
	GLUTEN-FREE OATS	1/2 PALM	1/3 CUP COOKED
	MILLET	1 PALM	1/3 CUP COOKED
BETTER	WHITE POTATO	1 PALM +	1/2 MEDIUM SIZE
	BLUEBERRIES	1 FIST	1 CUP
	RASPBERRIES	1 FIST +	1 ¼ CUPS
	AMARANTH	1 PALM	1/3 CUP COOKED
	BUCKWHEAT	1 PALM +	1/2 CUP COOKED
	BLACKBERRIES	1 FIST	1 ¼ CUPS
	CATALOUPE	2 FISTS	1 ½ CUPS, DICED
	ENGLISH MUFFIN (GLUTEN FREE)	N/A	1 SMALL
	WATERMELON	2 FISTS	1 ½ CUPS, DICED
	ORANGE	N/A	1 LARGE
	GRAPEFRUIT	N/A	1 MEDIUM
	TANGERINE	N/A	2 MEDIUM
	CRACKER(GLUTEN-FREE, WHOLE GRAIN)	8 SMALL	8 SMALL CRACKERS
	80-100% DARK CHOCOLATE		2 SQUARES
GOOD	BANANA	N/A	1 SMALL / ½ LARGE
	KIWI	N/A	2 MEDIUM
	PEACH	N/A	1 LARGE
	CARROTS	1 PALM CHOPPED	1 CUP CHOPPED
	CORN	1 PALM	1/2 CUP
	BREAD, GLUTEN-FREE (Ezekiel, sprouted etc.)	N/A	1 SLICE
	CEREAL, GLUTEN-FREE, LOW SUGAR	1 PALM	1 CUP
	CORN TORTILLA	N/A	1 SMALL
	PITA, GLUTEN FREE	N/A	1 SMALL

AngelCARBS

	FOOD CHOICE	QUICK MEASURE	EXACT MEASUREMENT
BEST	KALE	UNLIMITED	UNLIMITED
	SPINACH		
	BRUSSELS SPROUTS		
	BROCCOLI		
	COLLARD GREENS		
	LEAFY GREENS		
	ASPARAGUS		
	STRING BEANS		
	BOK CHOY		
BETTER	TOMATOES		
	SNOW PEAS		
	CABBAGE		
	CAULIFLOWER		
	ARTICHOKES		
	BELL PEPPERS		
	EGG PLANT		
	ARUGALA		
	PICKLES		
GOOD	CUCUMBERS		
	CELERY		
	ROMAINE LETTUCE		
	ONIONS		
	MUSHROOMS		
	LOW-SUGAR TOMATO SAUCE		
	SPROUTS		

FREE FOODS

You may enjoy any of the foods, seasonings, and sauces below in unlimited amounts to ramp up flavor in any of your meals at any time.

- MUSTARDS – Dijon, regular yellow
- HERBS & SPICES - any
- EXTRACTS – vanilla, almond, peppermint
- VINEGARS – regular white and apple cider vinegar   FISH SAUCE – any
- CITRUS – lemon, lime juice
- SAUCES – Green chili sauce, salsa, low-sodium soya sauce, reduced sugar ketchup, siracha, hot sauce, tobasco, fish sauce, oyster sauce, Worcestershire sauce, low-cal steak sauce
- LOW CAL SALAD DRESSING – not "low-fat" as they are loaded with
- sugar.
- HERBAL & BLACK TEA – any, don't add sugar
- NATURAL SWEETENERS – stevia, xylitol
- BLACK COFFEE

PART THERE: CINDERELLA'S TOP 10: FLAVOR PAIRING & WEIGHT LOSS COMBINATIONS

Welcome to probably the most important piece of information you'll find in this entire program.

The reason for placing this ultra-valuable list in "not-so-plain-sight" is because I want to reward those who have taken the time to read all of the material to get a complete and clear understanding of ALL the material that will not only fast-track you to your goal, but allow you to surpass that goal and hit other milestones for years to come.

These are the very same list of principles that my Cinderella research team extracted from the World's top bio-nutrition experts and expert level scientist in my quest to help women like us lose the weight and keep it off forever in the healthiest most efficient ways possible.

Even though most of these techniques are already built into the program itself, having them at your fingertips will give you the power to be even more flexible when it comes to food choices during the program and the knowledge needed to maintain the body we build together over the next few weeks.

Enjoy!

1. Cinnamon & Starches/Sugars

The evidence supporting Cinnamon's blood sugar regulating capabilities actually rival the power of prescription diabetes medication like Metphornin and Antagon.

Apart from the beneficial effects on insulin resistance, cinnamon can lower blood sugar by decreasing the amount of glucose that enters your bloodstream after a high-carb or sugar-rich meal by interfering with numerous digestive enzymes (good thing) slowing the breakdown of carbohydrates in your digestive tract.

Secondly, cinnamon can benefit cells by mimicking insulin itself thus improving glucose uptake.

Numerous human studies have confirmed the anti-diabetic effects of cinnamon, showing that it can lower fasting blood sugar levels by 10–29%

Put it in PLAY:

In order to get the benefits of the carbs you've been missing out on for so long, while eliminating any option to store them as fat, try to add a pinch of cinnamon to all the meals that feature "Power Carbs" like fruit, potatoes, rice etc.

Also do this prior to your cheat meals and if there is a time where you fall off track with candy, cake or any sugary indulgence. Get a glass of hot water with cinnamon in you as soon as possible to regulate blood sugar and prevent all the sugar from landing on that butt and tummy.

2. Coffee and Cocoa

This is by far one of the most powerful flavor-paring weapons you can use!

The regular consumption of cocoa controls fat-cell metabolism to reduce the absorption of fatty acids in your body. Besides aiding in reducing obesity, appropriate consumption of cocoa improves internal heat production (thermogenesis) in the liver and white adipose tissues.

Coffee on the other hand actually has the power to activate fat cells and mobilize them into your bloodstream to be used as energy.

This is why sprinkling a little cocoa powder in your coffee creates a supercharged fat-burning effect. While the cocoa has the ability to prevent the body from storing fat, the coffee helps free your fat cells to be burned faster.

Put it in PLAY:

In your morning coffee (free of fat-storing creams and milk) sprinkle in a pinch of pure cocoa powder to ramp up fat burning while preventing any fat accumulation. Remember cocoa has a little caffeine in it as well so try not to consume this beverage after 1pm so you can get your beauty sleep.

3. Carbs and Protein

This is one of my favorites that I used every day on my own journey.

If you've been trying to lose weight, there's a good chance you've been shying away from carbs for the last couple years Which is why you may have been pleasantly surprised to see all the carbs on your meal plans.

Although the meal planning is taken care of for you, it's important to know how to eat carbs to get all their benefits while eliminating any of the negative effects so I've gone into a little more detail on this one.

First let's figure out why you should be eating more carbs....

If you've been shying away from carbs, just remember, Carbohydrates are your body's main source of energy: They help fuel your brain, kidneys, heart, muscles and central nervous system. For instance, fiber is a carbohydrate that aids in digestion, helps you feel full and keeps blood cholesterol levels in check. The way your meal plans are designed to actually shuttle extra carbohydrates in your muscles and liver for energy rather than storing them as fat. The truth is, A carbohydrate-deficient diet may cause headaches, fatigue, weakness, difficulty concentrating, nausea, constipation, bad breath and vitamin and mineral deficiencies.

The problem is that most of us pair our carbs with the wrong types of foods or with nothing at all. Whether you eat a bowl of healthy rice or smashed sweet potato that has zero added sugar or reach for a chocolate bar or candy that's loaded with extra sugar, your body goes through similar processes. Within minutes your body spikes insulin to convert those healthy carbs into a form of sugar called glycogen that is used for energy. The problem is, the faster the conversion rate the more likely those carbs are going to end up as fat rather than being used as energy.

The key here is to slow down your body's insulin response. This is already taken care of for you in the program by selecting the most fibrous carbs on the planet

which cause an immediate slowdown. However, you can enhance this effect by including something that has the ability to manage blood sugar levels even more efficiently.

By adding healthy protein choices along with your power carbs, you increase your ability to prevent those carbs from getting stored as fat while increasing fat burning capabilities with the thermogenic effect of lean protein sources.

Put it in Play:

Remember, this is one of the key reasons why the Japanese eat twice as many carbs as any other country and stay so lean and healthy. Again, this is taken care of for you throughout the program, but I want this drilled into you for when you're all done: Never eat even healthy carbs by themselves. Think toast and jam, fruit by itself, grilled cheese sandwiches. For example, if you're going to have a bowl of pasta, make sure there is a lean "Prime-Protein" in there like chicken or even meatballs. If mashed potatoes are on the menu be sure there is a side of salmon etc. Don't worry about the increased calories – think about those extra Cals as insulin spike reducing, fat accumulation preventing nutrients that help you get leaner by actually eating more food .

4.Lemon and Apple Cider Vinegar

It seems like Apple cider vinegar (ACV) and lemon detoxes have been the "darling" of internet cleanses over the last few years. And there's good reason for it because when you list the proven detoxification benefits of both you end up with a duo that will have your insides looking spotless.

The problem with those 1, 3- and 5-day cleanses are not only that they have you guzzling gallons of lemon juice and ACV, but they inevitably come to an end. No directions for including them into your daily routine and almost more importantly, they never list all their other benefits including their ability to increase insulin sensitivity, mobilize fatty tissue for energy and enhanced mood and cognitive function.

Here's how it works:

ACV and lemons are high in potassium and acetic acid which stimulates brain and nerve function. When these two functions are not at their peak, you are more likely to cave into cravings. The brains key decision maker, the Pre-Frontal Cortex thrives when flooded with potassium which allows you to keep willpower functioning at optimal levels. And when you're intestinal lining is left spotless from the ACV's acetic acid; multiple studies show improved mood and decision making because of an improved "brain-gut" connection.

Combine all this with a boost in energy, craving suppression and heart health and from the pectin found in the lemons and the chlorogenic acid in the vinegar and you can never go wrong with this dynamic duo.

And although the two do produce an amplified synergistic effect when taken

together, there is no reason you can't find a few ways to squeeze them in on their

own separately which we'll get into now.

Put it in Play:

Try to include lemon into any meal you see fit. That means on fish, potatoes, rice and as a salad dressing base. Squeeze some into your water whenever you can to ramp-up taste and keep a steady stream of brain-enhancing, craving reducing nutrients flowing all day long

Lemon juice and AVC help to suppress your appetite and aids in digestion and alkalinity as well. By helping you feel fuller longer, so you don't end up overeating. Studies have shown that if you maintain a more alkaline diet you will lose weight faster. So do your best to use ACV as a base for the salad dressings that list vinegar as its base or even as a marinade base for some of your meats.

Finally, you can get this duo in you the most efficient way by adding a tiny dose to your water throughout the day. A few years ago, I wanted to see if I could stop drinking (and spending a ton of money) on coffee. When I dropped to coffee I added this ACV and lemon to the giant bottle of water that I promised myself that I'd drink each day on my coffee detox. After a few days I not only noticed improvement in mood and sleep, but I maintained consistent energy levels throughout the day without the coffee-crash!

5. Turmeric and Honey

While many of our flavor pairing rituals have been borrowed from the Japanese, this particular little gem is one that the Japanese borrowed from India. At first this may seem like an unusual pairing, and you're right, it is - but once you find out the benefits of this powerful combination you'll see why it made the list.

First turmeric on its own has been touted recently as one of the new miracle foods that the health and wellness community has latched onto over the last few years as a key anti-inflammatory miracle food. And since inflammation is not only related to increased rates of cancer, obesity, heart attack and especially brain related disease like dementia and Alzheimer's, it no wonder everyone's telling you to take it.

However, there is something that they're forgetting to tell you. While turmeric in its root and powder form on its own is very effective for digestive purposes, most promote turmeric itself as a key anti-inflammatory aid. The problem is and what they don't tell you is that the active ingredient needed to reduce inflammation, curcumin gets lost along the way. The most powerful part of this whole equation, the curcumin cannot cross the barrier needed to be absorbed by your blood, and thus most of us never get the cure-all effects!

What you need in order to get all the weight loss, anti-inflammatory and life- lengthening effects is a little Piperine and a 'controlled insulin pump, not a spike, just a little bump.

Put it in play

In order to get all the benefits of curcumin via the aforementioned delivery system (Piperine and increased insulin release) the answer is simple and delicious.

The way most Cinderella Success Stories make this happen is by having a mid-day soothing Turmeric-Pepper-Honey Tea. Although it may not sound super tasty, I'm sure you'll have no problem adding it to your daily routine after just one cup. The honey will add the tiny insulin release needed to absorb the Curcumin and the Piperine will act almost like a key unlocking the Piperine from the turmeric.

Instructions:

- Steep or boil 1 cup of water
- Add ½ teaspoon of turmeric powder
- 1 pinch of black pepper (preferably fresh ground)
- ½ tsp. honey

6. Fiber and Carbohydrates

Are you filling up on fiber? If you looking to lose weight while still enjoying the carbs you love, you should be!

Including high-fiber foods in your diet is a healthy and natural way to both while helping to reduced high blood sugar. As an added incentive, you will be able to stay full longer which is also going to help you knock off a couple bonus pounds as well.

Eating lots of fiber like the kind found in your Angel Carbs as well as the starchy carbs like rice and potatoes etc. found at the top of the "Power Carbs" list helps eliminate fat all over the body and specifically the deadly "visceral fat" that surrounds most of our organs!

Finally, if that wasn't enough, fiber promotes excellent bowel health, lowers the risk of cancer and heart disease while also controlling your blood sugar.

When fiber is digested, your body handles it differently than the way in which refined carbohydrates, such as white flour, are digested. A portion of the fiber simply passes through your digestive system intact. This difference means that eating foods rich in fiber eliminates any dramatic spikes in high blood sugar because fiber doesn't require insulin to digest, which also means that it can be counted against the total carbohydrates of that particular meal.

When you look at a nutrition facts table, you will typically find the suggested serving size at the top of the table and the grams of total carbohydrates per serving lower in the table. Below the total carbs, you will see the fiber content listed in grams. Fiber is accounted for as part of the total carbohydrates found in a food. In other words, it's listed twice -- once in the listing under "fiber" and once as part of the total carbohydrate count, which also includes starches and sugars.

For example, if a bowl of oatmeal has 30 grams of carbs but has 15 grams of fiber, you are only left with 15 total carbs that impact the body!

Put it in Play

Now, I've already given you recommendations on portion sizes and as I always say, I never want you to be a slave to calorie counting so I've taken care of a lot of this for you. All of your Power Carbs, specifically the top 10 on the list are chalked-full of fiber. And in those higher carbohydrate meals I recommend that you load up on angel carbs because those guys are fiber rich and will help with our goal of reducing total impact carbs.

However, this is real life and I know that sometimes you're not going to be able to

eat exactly what's on the Cinderella Menu, Right.

So, if you're out and about – or even when you're getting groceries have a look at your labels. If you are absolutely DYING for carbs, have a look at the label of the food you choose and look at the carb vs fiber amounts. If it's a higher carb option like a granola bar you won't feel guilty when you see that the fiber content is almost equal to the carbohydrates! That means you can sometimes have your cake and eat it too (as long as that cake has some fiber in it)

7.Zinc and Waking up

That's right one part of this equation is extremely easy – all you have to do is open those eyes and get your butt out of bed......the other part, the zinc part, isn't so simple....it not hard, but it's not simple either.

Zinc is a trace element that is absolutely essential for a healthy immune system. A lack of zinc can make a person more susceptible to disease and illness. This powerful little mineral is responsible for a number of functions in the human body, and it helps stimulate the activity of at least 100 different enzymes and the good news is a small intake of zinc is necessary to reap the benefits.

The bad news is that even getting a small amount of zinc in our body is a tough task. Most foods are low in zinc and most high-level zinc foods are also high carb foods as well - not that that's a bad thing, but in order to get the necessary amount of zinc needed to facilitate weight loss, immune function and better sleep, you would have to be eating a lot of carbs very often.

However, Eggs are a great choice! They have absolutely zero carbs and a large amount of zinc. they are an excellent choice!

Put it in play

As you will see we have already taken care of this for you in your meal plans by adding many meals that include eggs in one way or another. Whether it be as a baking ingredient in your lunches, dinners and snacks or in the more traditional forms of just having eggs for breakfast.

Not a fan of eggs? I'm with you! I never really was either and sometimes busy ladies like us don't have time to whip up eggs every morning.

If you're in that category, I've included the most naturally zinc rich foods in all of your morning meals. Plus, most fitness gurus recommend taking the best part out of the egg, the yolk, which happens to be the part of the egg that contains all the zinc.Once you have a look at some of the recipes provided, I think you'll agree that eggs are a pleasant tasty and nutritious way to start the day.

And if you're worried about cholesterol, the team has portioned out servings so that you are only getting the newly proven, doctor recommended, heart healthy serving of healthy cholesterol.

8.Olive oil and Salt

While both salt and olive oil make a welcome addition to almost any meal, I'm not talking about a flavor pairing you put in your mouth here. I want these 2 health and wellness powerhouses in your tub! Out of all the pairings and combinations listed this one definitely ranks in my top 3 not only for the proven scientific and biological benefits but for the way it makes me feel....immediately!

Let's get the "science-stuff" out of the way first.

Extra Virgin Olive oil contains vitamin E, anti-oxidants, and compounds such as squalene and oleocanthal which prevent aging and repair skin damage. Olive oil is non-toxic, anti-microbial, and hypoallergenic.

Plus, on top of that this is what the beautiful Sophia Lauren attributes to be the sole reason to her almost ageless existence. When asked how she stays looking so young well into her 80's she said: "my mother and sisters all looked old before their time, the only thing I did differently was something a friend's grandmother showed me in my teenage years. Whenever I draw a bath, I release one cap of olive oil into the water".

As for the second half of the equation, Salt, when adding it to your bath, most women prefer the Epsom Salt variety for its increased mineral properties, 21 to be exact, like magnesium, potassium, sodium, sulfur, zinc, calcium, chloride, iodide, and bromide, all of which work synergistically to nourish our bodies.

When it comes to weight loss specifically this combination adds a double-punch by adding a dual pulling effect drawing the toxins from the body that induce inflammation and prevent fat mobilization for energy. This itself leads to 3 other key ingredients 1) Reduce insomnia by increasing circulation and adding magnesium, a common ingredient in most sleep-aids 2) Relief of arthritis pain including osteoarthritis, rheumatoid arthritis, and psoriatic arthritis. And 3)

improving skin quality and relief from eczema. In one German study patients with active eczema soaked one arm in a Dead Sea salt solution and their other arm in tap water for 15 minutes a day for 6 weeks. Soaking in the Dead Sea salt solution significantly improved skin barrier function, hydration, and inflammation compared with the tap water-treated side.

Put it in Play:

Simply add 1 capful of olive oil and as much as one cup of Epsom salts to your warm bath. The more is better approach is NOT recommended here unless you want to step out of that bath feeling like a pork-chop ready for the grill.

And even with this minimal dose of each, be sure to towel off thoroughly. For the sake of anybody else who lives with you, maybe devote a special towel to your salty-oil bath as well.

Don't have time for a bath? Yes, you do. I don't want to be one of those people who say "make time" but....MAKE TIME. Light a candle, draw the bath, put in your "potion" and turn everything (and everyone) else off. This is your time, do something for you and relax. Speaking of relaxing, I almost forgot to mention....remember the whole "increased cortisol/stress thing keeping us ladies chubby?" A 10-minute warm bath (with or without salt and oil) has been proven to reduce blood pressure by 1o% and cortisol levels by 20.

Bottom Line....make time for yourself and your bath!

9.Ginger and Orange

As complex's and as efficient as the human body is, performing literally a million tasks at once, it still hasn't found out how to do everything, really well all at once. What I mean is, your body kind of has a "one track mind' and if its caught up doing one large task, some of the others will suffer. Especially when it comes to digestion.

Think of digestion as a workout for the entire inside of your body...

... Stomach acids are mobilized to break down food, the liver and kidneys jump in to eliminate toxin all while a few liters of blood are devoted to the whole process.

For many of us our digestive system has been experiencing an all-day traffic jam, even after the smallest meals which is one of the primary reasons most women have trouble losing weight or keeping it off. If the body is caught up with digesting and breaking down food, it cannot focus on our primary goal over the next few weeks of fat elimination and creating hormonal balance.

The ginger portion of this equation was lifted from our go to healthy country, Japan who eat ginger with almost every meal in its pickled form, while the citrus half was taken from the Germans who typically try to add oranges to almost each and every heavy meal.

This little root contains nine different substances that have been found to stimulate serotonin receptors in the gut which provide benefits to the gastrointestinal system, reducing gut-related inflammation and enhancing nutrient absorption.

Ginger is classified as a carminative (reducing intestinal gas) and an intestinal spasmolytic (soothes the intestinal tract), while inducing gut motility. Additionally, it helps aid in the production of bile, making it particularly helpful in digesting fats.

Ginger is classified as a carminative (reducing intestinal gas) and an intestinal spasmolytic (soothes intestinal tract) while inducing gut motility. Additionally, it helps aid in the production of bile, making it particularly helpful in digesting fats.

The other half of this equation, the citrus, specifically oranges takes care of the rest. For many of us even if our digestion is on track we fail when it comes to the most important part, nutrient and mineral absorption. Getting your hormones to work together to mobilize fat as fuel and takes a lot of help, or "ingredients" and oranges have them all.

While the heavy dose of vitamin C in any citrus fruit plays a key role in helping the gut and intestinal track absorb those precious nutrients, oranges perform best when it comes to assimilation of iron – a key fat mobilization and energy enhancing aid. Oranges take multitasking to the next level by promoting a "blunted" insulin spike that not only helps digest the food itself, but sooth insulin sensitivity as well.

Put it in play:

Option 1 (my go-to)

Almost every night before bed I treat myself to an "Orange Ginger Digestive" tea so my body can focus on burning fat while I sleep instead of devoting all its energy to digesting my last meal. While you may be able to find an orange ginger tea at the grocery store, I prefer to make my own just because I know I'm getting about 5-10 times the nutrients needed with the DIY version.

To make enough for a few cups later in the week or even better, a cold glass in the afternoon tomorrow, boil 4 cups of water with 1 inch of ginger sliced into tiny pieces along with one full orange sliced into circular slices. Add a natural sweetener if you like and let this powerful concoction go to work.

BTW: This is one of my favorite nighttime "craving-killers" as well!

10. Oxygen and H20

This combination is designed to flood the body, blood and brain with the primary elements that keep you alive.... makes sense, right?

We do this by ingesting massive doses of oxygen while reinvigorating its only means of transportation, your blood.

Again, cortisol and dehydration levels are naturally at their highest upon rising and in the midafternoon. Although you may not feel "stressed" or dehydrated when you wake up, your stress hormone is pumping in excess in order to get the rest of the body ready for action. And while you were snoozing, every piece and every cell went through a massive regeneration and renewal process which used a ton of your bodies water supply.

Mid-day, around 1-3 in the afternoon where cortisol and dehydration reach its second peak from less-evolutionary" means. For most of us we've already dealt with a bunch of micro-stressors that could stem from a number of bothersome or annoying situations and in the midst of all this you haven't drank the right amount of water to stay hydrated.

And the bottom line is, if your stress hormone is pumping and you're dehydrated the last thing your body is focused on is losing weight. In fact, the opposite is true; you're more likely to add pounds here as the body looks to save up fuel (fat and water) in case of emergency.

With all this in mind, it's time to use an easy yet proven technique that immediately suppresses cortisol and stress levels along with a cocktail that provides natural energy, rehydration, detoxification while alkalizing the body.

Put it in Play:

Ideally every morning and every afternoon when you can, you will practice 10-20 reps of breathwork for immediate cortisol reduction plus all day cortisol regulation and to improve Tissue Function & Prevention. All organs perform better when fully oxygenated plus most diseases cannot thrive in an optimally oxygenized environment. This will provide an immediate and prolonged stimulation of the lymphatic system.

This should be followed by drinking 1-16oz (250ml-500ml) of "alkalized water "this will cause a 20-24% boost in metabolic function, elimination of dehydration after 7-8 hours of sleep. You'll also Increase nutrient absorption and create an "Alkaline" environment in your body that provides clean energy, fat oxidization and mental focus using some of the principles borrowed from flavor-pairing #4 (lemon and ACV).

Breathwork Technique

1 REP EQUALS:

- Take a deep breath in through the nose that lasts 4 seconds.
- Hold your breath for two seconds.
- Exhale from the nose and mouth "through the diaphragm" for 5-6 seconds releasing every last bit of air.
- During these repetitions focus on nothing but your breathing. This may be tough to do at first. Thoughts will enter your mind but simply recognize that thought, dismiss it and refocus on your breathing.

X15-20 repetitions

Alkalized Water INGREDIENTS*:

WATER: 500ml/16.9 fl oz (minimum) LEMON JUICE: ½ squeezed lemon

1 pinch of baking soda or sea salt

Look at you!!!!!

You've just completed the C.S. Main Book and Owner's Manual. If you're reading this page, you are either on the edge of starting this incredible journey or you decided to jump in head-first with the C.S. Quick Start Guide and you are already a couple days in to this.

Either way I truly cannot wait for you to start this incredible transformation. As I write this, I'm looking out my office window. It's the same desk and the same computer that I crafted my original weight loss ritual book that I used to lose almost 100 pounds.

I remember sitting here back then so desperate for change, finding these secrets in buried medical journals, after talking to doctors on the other side of the world and saying to myself....this just might work.

I had never had that kind of peace of mind when I tried to lose weight in the past. What gets me a little sappy is thinking about the fact that your fate is now sealed as well....just like mine was when I first started. THIS IS GOING TO WORK, and this WILL BE THE LAST TIME YOU EVER HAVE TO LOSE WEIGHT.

Just like Cinderella, you've now got that glass slipper that opened up a whole new world for her.... it's in your hands...now all you've gotta do is put it on and start charging toward that brand new you!

QUICK START

Cinderella Solution QUICK START

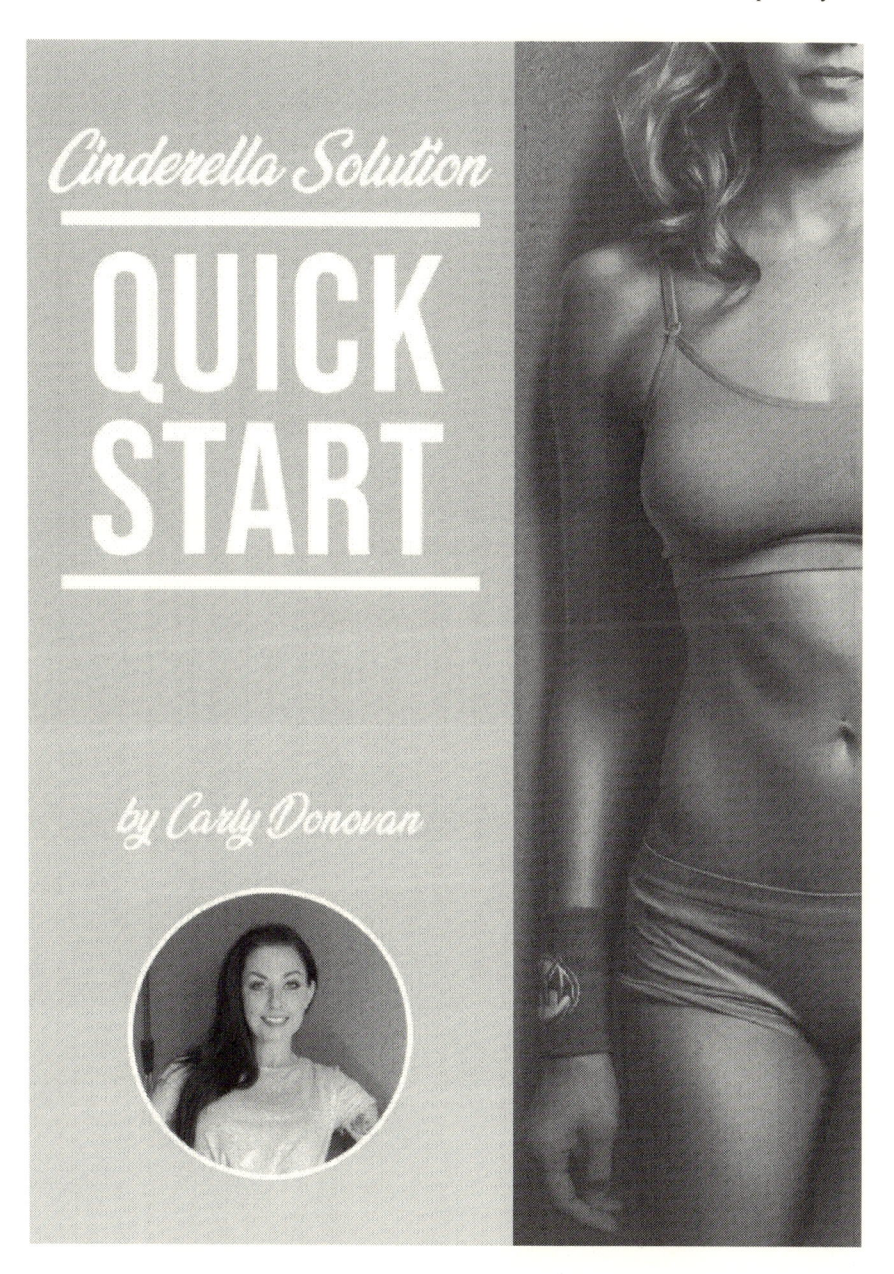

by Carly Donovan

How Exciting!

Just think: This is it.

This is the last time you will ever have to try to lose weight. It's a pretty exciting feeling, right? No more starving yourself on diets that don't work or workout routines that have you exercising for hours at a time...

Never again.

You are FINALLY going to experience what it looks, and most importantly feels like, when you permanently banish all the fat that has slowly crept around your tummy, waist, hips and legs over the years.

The best part is, by the time you are done you will have completely transformed your metabolism making rebound weight gain almost impossible.

Ask any Cinderella Success Story what the best part of finally building their dream body is and you will be shocked to hear that it's NOT all the weight they lost.

Although rapid, safe and permanent weight loss is inevitable on the Cinderella plan, the biggest gift you will receive by the time you are done is control.

As the original Cinderella Success Story, I promise you, words cannot describe what it feels like to finally be in control of how you look and feel every single day.

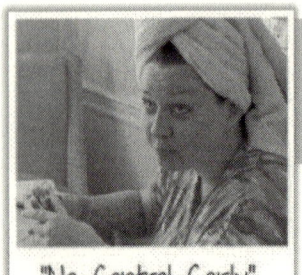

"No-Control-Carly"

I know sometimes it can feel like you've lost control of your own body.

I used to be controlled by my reflection in the mirror and it would send my confidence into the gutter every single day. My weight controlled the social situations I attended by making me wonder who was going to be there, and if I wanted them to see me after gaining all the weight. I even felt controlled by what I wore... I would cut any tag off the clothes that had an "L" or "XL" on them, because just knowing those tags were on there made me feel ashamed.

I know to some of you that may sound extreme, but if you are reading this, then I know you have a motivation deeper than simply "losing a couple pounds".

This is where I want you to dig deep and figure out your real "why".

Whatever your motivation may be, whether it is getting back the energy you had when you were a kid, or spending more time on this planet with your kids...

I'm here to tell you, you're in the right place and we are about to make that happen together.

Without further ado, let's get started on your very last weight loss journey and get empowered with all the information needed to regain control, while creating the body of your dreams.

For the "Start NOW, learn later" ladies...

Alright, if you are reading this book first, then you're in a hurry to get started. However, I just want you to know, no matter when you begin the Cinderella Solution, the weight is going to come off quickly!

Whether it's tomorrow or next week, your scale will be shooting out numbers that are going to put an all-day smile on your face.

However, in order to keep those pounds rolling off and keep them off forever, it's important to educate yourself on how weight-loss from the inside-out really works...

... With that in mind, go through this Quick Start Guide and get started as soon as you like – but PLEASE, PLEASE, PLEASE take advantage of all the Cinderella Resources in the full package when you have the time.

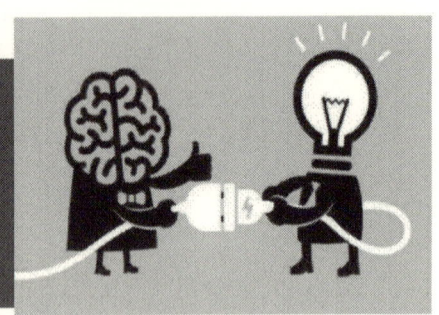

Of course, we designed this system so all you really need to get started is this book.

But if you just got your program and you want to get started burning fat as soon as tonight, be sure to empower yourself with all the information needed to lose the weight FASTER AND FOREVER by going through the Cinderella Solution Main Book & Owner's Manual too.

When you get a chance, read through the rest of the material to get a complete perspective on why you are doing this, how it works and most importantly why it works so darn well! Your chances of success will not only increase significantly, but you will be able to execute with purpose and precision every step of the way.

You will find on your journey that everybody likes to pretend they are the "expert" on the subject of getting in shape. Once you are schooled on how your body and getting in shape actually works, you will be able to put the "know-it-alls" in their place and maybe even help some of them along the way.

OK... Now You Can "Quick Start"

These Quick-Start Instructions will give you a basic understanding of how your programs works. I have done my best to ensure this book alone is as self-explanatory as possible.

If you are looking for more detail be sure to read the Cinderella Solution Main Book & Owner's Manual.

USING THE LAUNCH & IGNITE PHASES

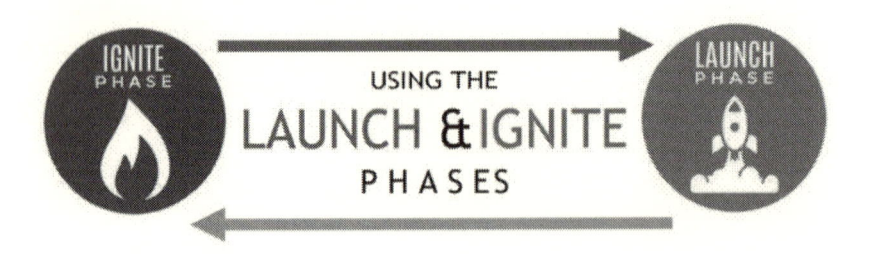

The Cinderella Solution consists of two 14-day phases:

"Ignite" and "Launch"

The first 2-week phase, "Ignite", is specifically designed to act as a cleansing detoxification that not only promotes fat loss, but re-ignites your fat burning hormones.

- Unlike traditional cleanses, you won't have to starve yourself and deprive your body of the vitamins and nutrients that actually heal your hormones. Instead, you will consume fat-fighting foods that target the trouble spots around your hips, butt, and belly in a format that resets and "re-ignites" your metabolism.
- In the Ignite Phase, you will skip the starchy "power carbs" at breakfast to promote a 15 to 18-hour total fat-burning flush that starts from dinner the night before and lasts all the way until lunch the next day!
- You will boost all your primary weight loss hormones (Insulin, Cortisol and Estrogen) by eliminating foods that harm and increasing the foods that help.

During this 14-day phase, you will re-train insulin sensitivity by forcing your body to use fat for fuel, down-regulate your stress hormone cortisol for belly-fat elimination, and improve digestion for the purging of fat- binding and excess estrogen containing molecules.

The second phase, "Launch" is designed to take weight-loss into overdrive by taking advantage of your body's newly enhanced hormonal and metabolic environment.

- With a totally "reset" metabolism, we can now re-introduce some of your favorite foods while increasing the carbs you crave. Expect explosive energy and an all-day feeling of wellbeing while your body continues to burn fat at an accelerated rate.
- Foods that may have caused weight gain in the past will actually help you unleash fat from all your trouble spots after priming your endocrine system during the Ignite Phase.
- We will introduce a brand-new nutrient and vitamin profile complete with Cinderella "flavor-pairing" rituals and "food combinations". Your body is a pretty smart machine and it can get-wise to the same old tricks if used over and over, which is why we keep the metabolism "on-its-toes" during the Launch Phase.

Cycling the Ignite & Launch Phases

You will start your program in the Ignite Phase first for 14 days, followed by the Launch Phase for another 14 days.

If you haven't lost all the weight you feel you have to lose after completing the 2 phases (28 days total), then simply begin again in Ignite for 2 weeks followed by another 2 weeks of Launch. Follow this sequence until you reach your total weight-loss goal.

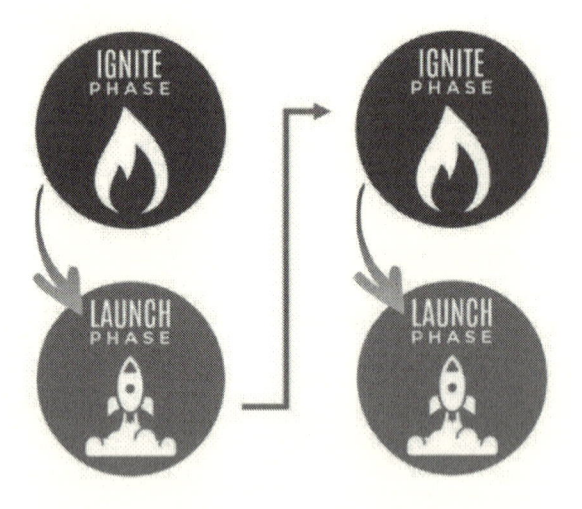

For more information on Cinderella's two-phase IGNITE & LAUNCH system and why it works so well, read chapter 3 inside the Cinderella Solution Main Book and Owner's Manual

Alright, Get Going Girl!

Below are a couple of last-minute notes before you begin the program:

- [x] You can choose to follow the done-for-you plan or create your own meals using the food lists!

- [x] Review your grocery list based on your done for you meals and have a look at some of the key Weight Loss Rituals like the Flavor-Pairings & Food Combinations and prep some of the staples in advance for convenience.

- [x] When you get a chance, start reading the "Cinderella Main Book & Owner's Manual" so you can understand the detailed explanations and tips to lose weight even faster, as well as clearing up absolutely any other question you may have.

Cinderella Solution

Cinderella Solution
"DO-IT-YOURSELF" MEAL CREATOR & FLAVOR PAIRING

IGNITE & LAUNCH MEAL LEGENDS

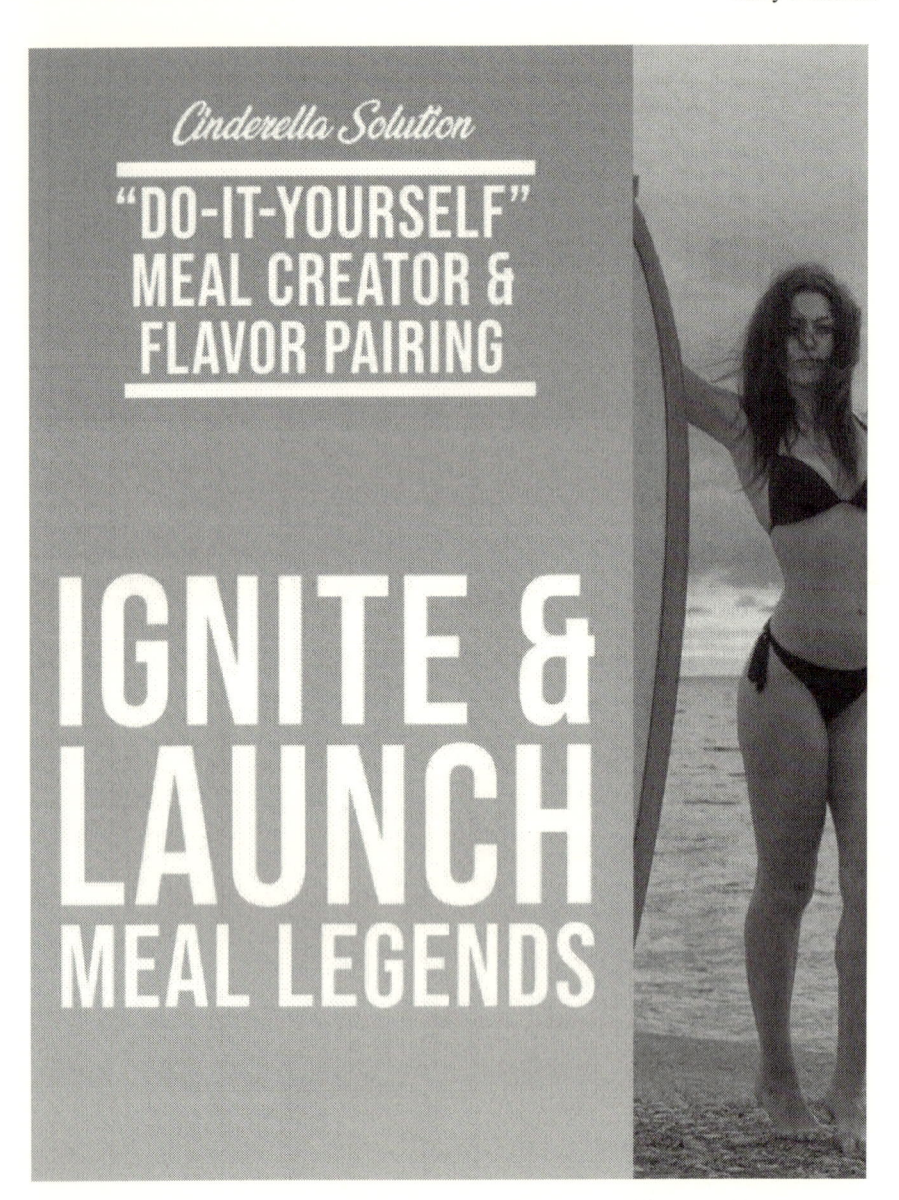

Making Your Own Meals

These are the Food-Pairing Legends you will use during the Ignite and Launch Phases to create your meals. The corresponding food blocks/portions with food choices for Prime Proteins, Royal Fats,

Power Carbs and Angel Carbs are below:

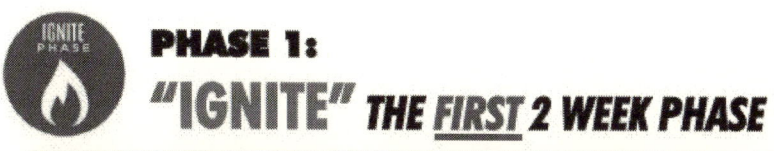

PHASE 1:
"IGNITE" THE FIRST 2 WEEK PHASE

IGNITE PAIRINGS

MEAL	PRIME PROTEIN	ROYAL FAT	POWER CARB	ANGEL CARB
BREAKFAST	2	2	0	UNLIMITED
LUNCH	2	1	2	UNLIMITED
DINNER	2	2	0	UNLIMITED

PHASE 2:
"LAUNCH" THE SECOND 2 WEEK PHASE

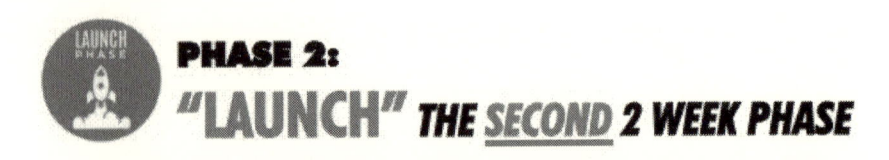

LAUNCH PAIRINGS

MEAL	PRIME PROTEIN	ROYAL FAT	POWER CARB	ANGEL CARB
BREAKFAST	1	1	1	UNLIMITED
LUNCH	1	2	0	UNLIMITED
SNACK*	1 OR	1 +	1	UNLIMITED (optional)
DINNER	2	2	0	UNLIMITED

*Remember, your "LAUNCH" snack includes 1 POWER CARB combined with either 1 ROYAL FAT or 1 PRIME PROTEIN

Also, your second POWER CARB meal can be at Lunch or Snack time — they are interchangeable based on your preference. You can see examples of how this is done on your sample "Launch Meals" plan

EXAMPLE IGNITE MEAL CREATION

FOR EXAMPLE

In your IGNITE BREAKFAST Food Legend, you are asked to have:

2 PRIME PROTEINS, 2 ROYAL FATS, 0 POWER CARBS

MEAL	PRIME PROTEIN	ROYAL FAT	POWER CARB	ANGEL CARB
BREAKFAST	2	2	0	UNLIMITED

Say you would like to make an omelette for breakfast, all you have to do is simply refer to the Food Block/Portion pages that follow and build your meal. Portion sizes for "Free Hand" measurement and "The Weigh Way" are both listed to make everything super quick and really easy.

PRIME PROTEIN	ROYAL FAT	POWER CARB	ANGEL CARB
2 =	2 =	0 =	UNLIMITED
2/3 C. EGG WHITES	1 WHOLE EGG + 1 TBSP OLIVE OIL	N/A	MUSHROOMS & RED PEPPER

Although there are prescribed amounts and types of "Angel Carbs" in your meal plan, you may have as much of that vegetable/angel carb as you like.

Also keep in mind, that you can substitute any Angel Carb listed in the meal plans with any of the other Angel Carbs/Vegetables featured on the Angel Carbs list below.

Prime PROTEINS

BEST

FOOD CHOICE	QUICK MEASURE	EXACT MEASUREMENT
SARDINES	1/2 PALM	2 OZ. (2 MEDIUM SIZED)
BONELESS SKINLESS CHICKEN	1 PALM+	2 OZ. COOKED / 3 OZ RAW
EGG WHITES	N/A	3 LARGE OR 1/3 CUP
ANCHOVIES	1 PALM	3 OZ.
PROTEIN POWDER	N/A	1 TBSP (ROUNDED)
WHITE FISH (COD, TILAPIA ETC)	1 PALM+	3 OZ. COOKED / 4 OZ. RAW
SALMON/TUNA	1 PALM	2 OZ. COOKED / 3 OZ. RAW
GAME MEAT	1 PALM	2 OZ. COOKED / 3 OZ. RAW
GROUND TURKEY OR CHICKEN	1 PALM	2 OZ. COOKED / 3 OZ. RAW
RED MEAT (EXTRA LEAN)	1 PALM	2 OZ. COOKED / 3 OZ RAW

BETTER

FOOD CHOICE	QUICK MEASURE	EXACT MEASUREMENT
LOX, SALMON	½ PALM	2 OZ. RAW
ALMOND MILK	N/A	1 CUP
TURKEY BACON	N/A	2 SLICES
PORK TENDERLOIN	1 PALM	2 OZ. COOKED / 3 OZ RAW
SKINLESS CHICKEN THIGH/DRUM	1 PALM	2 OZ COOKED / 3 OZ. RAW
TURKEY/HAM SLICES, DELI	1 PALM	3 OZ. / 2 SLICES
TURKEY BREAKFAST SAUSAGE	N/A	1 SAUSAGE
GROUND BEEF, EXTRA LEAN	1 PALM	2 OZ. RAW / 3 OZ. COOKED
CLAMS/MUSSELS/SHRIMP	1 FIST	4 OZ. COOKED / 6 OZ RAW

VEGAN & VEGETARIAN (and super-picky eater) OPTIONS

While the animal-friendly options below are healthy, foods that contain dairy and soy in larger amounts can impede hormonal function and thus, weight loss. Feel free to use these options, but be sure to use them sparingly.

GOOD

FOOD CHOICE	QUICK MEASURE	EXACT MEASUREMENT
GREEK YOGURT	3/4 FIST	3/4 CUP
COTTAGE CHEESE	1 PALM	1/2 CUP
VEGGIE BURGER	N/A	1 SMALL PATTY (3 OZ.)
TEMPEH	1 PALM	2 OZ.
TOFU, EXTRA FIRM	1 PALM	3 OZ.
VEGGGIE-BACON	N/A	2 SLICES (1 OZ.)

Royal FATS

	FOOD CHOICE	QUICK MEASURE	EXACT MEASUREMENT
BEST	AVOCADO	2 THUMBS	1/4 SMALL-MEDIUM AVOCADO
	ALMONDS	1 THUMB	1 TBSP. CHOPPED/6 WHOLE
	CASHEWS	1 THUMB	1 TBSP. CHOPPED/4 WHOLE
	PUMPKIN SEEDS	1 THUMB+	2 TBSP.
	PECANS	1 THUMB	1 TBSP. CHOPPED/5 HALVES
	CHIA SEEDS	1 THUMB	2 ½ TSP.
	PISTACIOS	1 THUMB	1 TBSP. CHOPPED/10 WHOLE
	FLAX SEEDS, GROUND	1 THUMB	1 TBSP.
	SUNFLOWER SEEDS	1 THUMB	1 TBSP.
	SESAME SEEDS	1 THUMB	1 TBSP.
BETTER	EXTRA-VIRGIN OLIVE OIL	1 FOREFINGER TIP	1 TSP
	CHIA OIL	1 FOREFINGER TIP	1 TSP
	1 WHOLE EGG	N/A	1 SMALL
	ALMOND BUTTER	1 FOREFINGER TIP	1 ½ TSP.
	CASHEW BUTTER	1 FOREFINGER TIP	1 ½ TSP.
	PUMPKIN SEED OIL	1 FOREFINGER TIP	1 TSP
	COCONUT OIL/BUTTER	1 FOREFINGER TIP	1 TSP
	SHREDDED COCONUT, UNSWEET	2 THUMBS	2 TBSP
	COCONUT MILK, CANNED	2 THUMBS	5 TSP

VEGAN & VEGETARIAN (and super-picky eater) **OPTIONS**

While the animal-friendly options below are healthy, foods that contain dairy and soy in larger amounts can impede hormonal function and thus, weight loss. Feel free to use these options, but be sure to use them sparingly.

	FOOD CHOICE	QUICK MEASURE	EXACT MEASUREMENT
GOOD	FETA CHEESE	2 THUMBS	2 LEVEL TBSP.
	GOAT CHEESE	2 THUMBS	2 LEVEL TBSP.
	REAL MOZZARELLA	1 THUMB	2 LEVEL TBSP
	PARMESAN CHEESE (low sodium)	2 THUMBS	2 LEVEL TBSP. GRATED

Power CARBS

	FOOD CHOICE	QUICK MEASURE	EXACT MEASUREMENT
BEST	QUINOA	1 PALM	1/3 CUP COOKED
	WHITE OR BROWN RICE	1 PALM	1/3 CUP COOKED
	WILD RICE	1 PALM	1/3 CUP COOKED
	BEETS	N/A	2 MEDIUM
	PARSNIP	1 FIST MASHED	1 MEDIUM SIZE
	SWEET POTATO	1 FIST MASHED	1/2 MEDIUM SIZE
	SQUASH	2 FISTS	2 CUPS CUBED
	APPLES	N/A	1 SMALL
	PEARS	N/A	1 SMALL
	GLUTEN-FREE OATS	1/2 PALM	1/3 CUP COOKED
	MILLET	1 PALM	1/3 CUP COOKED
BETTER	WHITE POTATO	1 PALM +	1/2 MEDIUM SIZE
	BLUEBERRIES	1 FIST	1 CUP
	RASPBERRIES	1 FIST +	1 ¼ CUPS
	AMARANTH	1 PALM	1/3 CUP COOKED
	BUCKWHEAT	1 PALM +	1/2 CUP COOKED
	BLACKBERRIES	1 FIST	1 ¼ CUPS
	CATALOUPE	2 FISTS	1 ½ CUPS, DICED
	ENGLISH MUFFIN (GLUTEN FREE)	N/A	1 SMALL
	WATERMELON	2 FISTS	1 ½ CUPS, DICED
	ORANGE	N/A	1 LARGE
	GRAPEFRUIT	N/A	1 MEDIUM
	TANGERINE	N/A	2 MEDIUM
	CRACKERS (GLUTEN-FREE, WHOLE GRAIN)	8 SMALL	8 SMALL CRACKERS
	80-100% DARK CHOCOLATE		2 SQUARES
GOOD	BANANA	N/A	1 SMALL / ½ LARGE
	KIWI	N/A	2 MEDIUM
	PEACH	N/A	1 LARGE
	CARROTS	1 PALM CHOPPED	1 CUP CHOPPED
	CORN	1 PALM	1/2 CUP
	BREAD, GLUTEN-FREE (Ezekiel, sprouted etc.)	N/A	1 SLICE
	CEREAL, GLUTEN-FREE, LOW SUGAR	1 PALM	1 CUP
	CORN TORTILLA	N/A	1 SMALL
	PITA, GLUTEN FREE	N/A	1 SMALL

Angel **CARBS**

	FOOD CHOICE	QUICK MEASURE	EXACT MEASUREMENT
BEST	KALE	UNLIMITED	UNLIMITED
	SPINACH		
	BRUSSELS SPROUTS		
	BROCCOLI		
	COLLARD GREENS		
	LEAFY GREENS		
	ASPARAGUS		
	STRING BEANS		
	BOK CHOY		
	TOMATOES		
BETTER	SNOW PEAS		
	CABBAGE		
	CAULIFLOWER		
	ARTICHOKES		
	BELL PEPPERS		
	EGG PLANT		
	ARUGALA		
	PICKLES		
	CUCUMBERS		
GOOD	CELERY		
	ROMAINE LETTUCE		
	ONIONS		
	MUSHROOMS		
	LOW-SUGAR TOMATO SAUCE		
	SPROUTS		

As you move forward through this guide and into the meal plans, please remember that although there are prescribed amounts and types of "Angel Carbs" in your meal plan, you may have as much of that vegetable/angel carb as you like AND you can substitute them for any Angel Carb listed on this page!

FREE FOODS

You may enjoy any of the foods, seasonings, and sauces below in unlimited amounts to ramp up flavor in any of your meals at any time.

- MUSTARDS – Dijon, regular yellow   HERBS & SPICES - any
- EXTRACTS – vanilla, almond, peppermint
- VINEGARS – regular white and apple cider vinegar   FISH SAUCE – any
- CITRUS – lemon, lime juice
- SAUCES – Green chili sauce, salsa, low-sodium soya sauce, reduced sugar ketchup, siracha, hot sauce, tobasco, fish sauce, oyster sauce, Worcestershire sauce, low-cal steak sauce
- LOW CAL SALAD DRESSING – not "low-fat" as they are loaded with sugar.
- HERBAL & BLACK TEA – any, don't add sugar
- NATURAL SWEETENERS – stevia, xylitol   BLACK COFFEE

And as always, you can enjoy "Angel Carbs" in unlimited amounts at any time throughout the day!

IGNITE MEALS

DAY 1

Almond & Chia Protein Smoothie

Breakfast
7:00 AM

whey protein powder	1 Scoop
vanilla almond milk unsweetened	1 Cup(s)
almond butter, no salt	1 1/2 tsp
seeds chia dried	1 oz

Chicken Quinoa Medley

Lunch
12:00 PM

drinking water	2 Cup(s)
baby bok choy	1 cup raw
chicken breast, cooked	4 oz
extra virgin olive oil	2 Tbsp
quinoa, cooked	1 Cup(s)

Salmon Avocado Salad
(recipe pg. 22)

Dinner
6:00 PM

drinking water	2 Cup(s)
salmon avocado salad	1 serving

DAY 2

Omelet

Breakfast
7:00 AM

whole eggs, scrambled	2 large
drinking water	2 Cup(s)
asparagus, boiled	2 spears
mozzarella soy cheese, sliced	1 slice
olive oil	2 Tbsp

Taco Bowl

Lunch
12:00 PM

iced tea, green	2 Cup(s)
romaine lettuce	1 Cup(s)
ground turkey, cooked	4 oz
green chili peppers, canned	1/2 Tbsp
salsa, ready to serve	1/2 Tbsp
olive oil	1 Tbsp
brown rice, cooked	1 Cup(s)

Korean BBQ Keto Bowl
(recipe pg. 22)

Dinner
6:00 PM

drinking water	2 Cup(s)
korean bbq keto bowl	1/2 serving
baby bok choy	1/2 cup raw
coconut vegetable oil	1 Tbsp

DAY 3

Salmon Avocado Egg Wrap
(recipe pg. 23)

Breakfast
7:00 AM

drinking water	2 Cup(s)
salmon & avocado, keto egg wrap	1/2 serving
bacon, low-sodium, cooked	3 slice cooked

Tuna Sandwich

Lunch
12:00 PM

tuna fish, very low-sodium, in water	5 oz
drinking water	2 Cup(s)
asparagus, boiled	6 spears
ezekiel 4:9 sprouted 100% whole grain bread by foo...	2 slice
olive oil	2 Tbsp
lemon juice	1 1 wedge

Pork Chop & Veggies

Dinner
6:00 PM

drinking water	2 Cup(s)
baked pork chops (paleo)	1 serving
broccoli, no salt, steamed	2 Cup(s)
dairy free butter by vitalite	1 serving
cauliflower, no salt, boiled	1 Cup(s)

DAY 4

Creamy Almond Smoothie

Breakfast
7:00 AM

whey protein powder	1 Scoop
almond butter, no salt	1 Tbsp
pure vanilla almond milk unsweetened by silk	1 1/2 Cup(s)
avocado	1/2 avocado

Shrimp Stir-Fry

Lunch
12:00 PM

baby bok choy	1/4 cup raw
iced tea, green	2 Cup(s)
bamboo shoots raw	1/4 cup (1/2" pieces)
sesame oil, salad or cooking	1 Tbsp
shrimp, cooked	4 oz
brown rice, cooked	1 Cup(s)

Roasted Turkey Breast & Veggies

Dinner
6:00 PM

drinking water	2 Cup(s)
olive oil	1 1/2 Tbsp
swiss chard, no salt, boiled	1/2 cup, chopped
turkey breast, roasted	6 oz

DAY 5

Grab-and-Go Breakfast

Breakfast
7:00 AM

egg, hard boiled	2 large
drinking water	2 Cup(s)
cheddar cheese	1/4 oz
american soy cheese, sliced	2 slice
red peppers	1 cup, chopped

Turkey Quinoa Salad

Lunch
12:00 PM

turkey breast, roasted	4 oz
soybean mayonnaise salad dressing, no salt	1 1/2 tbsp
quinoa, cooked	1 Cup(s)
swiss chard, no salt, boiled	2 cup, chopped

Zucchini Noodle Shrimp Scampi
(recipe pg. 24)

Dinner
6:00 PM

drinking water	2 Cup(s)
zucchini noodle shrimp scampi	1 serving
parmesan cheese, grated	2 Tbsp

DAY 6

Mexican Breakfast Skillet

Breakfast
7:00 AM

drinking water	1 Cup(s)
egg whites, cooked	4 large
ground turkey, cooked	1 oz
olive oil	1 Tbsp
salsa, ready to serve	1/2 Tbsp
avocado	1/2 avocado

Halibut & Sweet Potato

Lunch
12:00 PM

drinking water	2 Cup(s)
baby bok choy	1/4 cup raw
bamboo shoots raw	1/4 cup (1/2" pieces)
sweet potato, no salt, baked	1 medium
olive oil	1 Tbsp
halibut fish, cooked	4 oz

Leftover Shrimp Scampi (day 5)

Dinner
6:00 PM

drinking water	2 Cup(s)
zucchini noodle shrimp scampi	1 serving
parmesan cheese, grated	2 Tbsp

DAY 7

Kale and Honey Protein Smoothie
(recipe pg. 25)

Breakfast
7:00 AM

drinking water	2 Cup(s)
whey protein powder	1 Scoop
avocado	1/2 avocado
pure vanilla almond milk unsweetened by silk	1 Cup(s)
kale	1 cup, chopped
cucumber, peeled	1/2 medium
honey	1 Tbsp

Pork Chop, Salad & Quinoa

Lunch
12:00 PM

romaine lettuce	4 leaf
italian spiced pork chops (paleo)	1 serving
quinoa, cooked	1 Cup(s)

Sage & Garlic Roasted Chicken
(recipe pg. 26)

Dinner
6:00 PM

sage & garlic roasted chicken	1 serving

1 Servings

ginger turmeric smoothie

Ingredients

bananas	1/2 extra large
pineapple	1/2 Cup(s)
ginger root	1 tsp
spices turmeric ground	1/4 tsp
lemon juice	1 Tbsp
honey	1 tsp
coconut milk beverage, unsweetened	1 Cup(s)

Instructions

1. Place all ingredients in blender.
2. Add approx. 1 cup of ice - add more if you desire a thicker smoothie.
3. Blend thoroughly until all ingredients are pureed. Drink immediately.

1 Servings

salmon avocado salad

Ingredients

white wine vinegar	1 Tbsp
coriander/ cilantro/ chinese parsley	2 tsp
green leaf lettuce	1 1/2 cup shredded
cherry tomatoes	6 tomatoes
olive oil	1/3 Tbsp
avocados	1/4 avocado
salmon, cooked	4 oz
mushrooms	1/8 cup, pieces or slices

Instructions

1. Preheat the oven broiler. Line a baking sheet with aluminum foil. Place the salmon on the foil. Season with salt and pepper. Broil 15 minutes, until fish is easily flaked with a fork.

2. Saute the mushrooms until tender.

2. Place the tomatoes in a bowl, and drizzle with 1 tablespoon olive oil. Season with salt and pepper.

3. In a large bowl, toss together the salmon, mushrooms, tomatoes, lettuce, avocado, cilantro. Drizzle with remaining olive oil and the vinegar. Season with salt and pepper, and sprinkle with feta cheese if desired, to serve.

4 Servings

korean bbq keto bowl

Ingredients

sriracha, hot chili sauce	2 Tbsp
ginger, ground	1/2 Tbsp
garlic	1 clove
coconut vegetable oil	2 Tbsp
cauliflower	1 head, small (4" dia)
cilantro leaves raw, coriander	1 Tbsp
skirt steak, lean	16 oz

Instructions

1. Mix sriracha, ginger and garlic for the marinade in a gallon sized sealable bag.
2. Place the sliced steak in the bag with the marinade and make sure the steak is well-coated.
3. Marinade for a minimum of 1 hour; recommended to marinade overnight.
4. Heat coconut oil in a large nonstick skillet. Add cauliflower (riced cauliflower recommended). Cook cauliflower until tender.
5. Heat a large cast iron skillet or grill pan on high heat until very hot.
6. Grill steak in batches, cooking until desired doneness.
7. Place steak over prepared cauliflower; garnish with minced fresh cilantro and serve.

2 Servings

salmon & avocado, keto egg wrap

Ingredients

egg	3 egg
avocados	1/2 avocado
fish salmon chinook smoked	2 oz, boneless
cream cheese	2 Tbsp
chives	2 tsp chopped
butter, no salt	1 Tbsp
black pepper	2 dash
green onions/scallions	1 tbsp chopped

Instructions

1. Crack the eggs into a mixing bowl and whisk. Add in black pepper.
2. In a small bowl, combine cream cheese and sliced chives.
3. Melt butter in a medium sized omelette pan. Pour in whisked eggs.
4. Cook omelette until soft, yet cooked through.
5. Slide the omelette onto a plate and top with cream cheese/chive mixture.
6. Top with sliced avocado, smoked salmon and green onions.
7. Fold the omelette into a wrap.

4 Servings

baked pork chops (paleo)

Ingredients

paprika	1/2 tsp
sage, ground	1/2 tsp
pork tenderloin	16 oz
vegetable oil, canola	2 Tbsp

Instructions

1. Combine spices in small bowl.

2. Rub spice mixture onto each side of raw pork chop.

3. Heat canola oil over medium-high heat; add pork chops.

4. While pork chops are browning; preheat oven to 425 degrees F.

5. Once each side of the pork chops are browned (not cooked through), transfer to oven safe dish and cover with foil. Bake until cooked through.

2 Servings

zucchini noodle shrimp scampi

Ingredients

zucchini/summer squash	2 medium
olive oil	2 Tbsp
shrimp	16 oz
garlic	1 clove
butter, no salt	2 Tbsp
parsley	2 tsp
crushed red pepper flakes	1 tsp
white wine	1 Tbsp
lemon juice	1 Tbsp

Instructions

1. Cut zucchini into noodles, using a mandoline or a spiralizer. Set aside.
2. Place a large sauté pan over medium heat. Add the olive oil and heat.
3. Add the garlic and crushed red pepper flakes, stirring constantly.
4. Add the shrimp to the pan, stirring as needed, until they are cooked through.
5. Use a slotted spoon to remove shrimp from pan. Set aside.
6. Leave remaining liquid in pan. Increase heat to medium-high. Add in white wine, lemon juice and butter.
7. Cook until sauce has reduced and thickened slightly. Add the zucchini noodles and cook for 2 minutes, or until tender.
8. Toss in prepared shrimp and garnish with minced fresh parsley.

1 Servings

italian spiced pork chops (paleo)

Ingredients

pork tenderloin	7 oz
sage, ground	1/4 tsp
onions	1/2 cup, sliced

Instructions

1. Preheat oven to 425°.

2. In a small bowl, mix the, pepper, paprika, and sage together.

3. Sprinkle both sides of each pork chop with the seasoning mixture.

4. Add lard to a skillet over high heat.

5. When good and hot, brown both sides of each chop.

6. Place the browned chops on a large piece of heavy foil and layer with sliced onions.

7. Close the foil into a tight pouch and place on a baking sheet.

8. Bake for 30 minutes, or until pork reaches desired temperature.

1 Servings

sage & garlic roasted chicken

Ingredients

sage, ground	1 tsp
olive oil	1 Tbsp
black pepper	1 tsp
garlic powder	1 tsp
chicken breast, boneless skinless	5 oz

Instructions

Preheat oven to 375. Wash chicken inside and out, pat dry with paper towels. In a small bowl, whisk together sage, oil, garlic and pepper. Rub this mixture under the skin of the breast and on the skin all over the chicken. Place chicken, breast side down, on lightly greased pan. Roast for 30 minutes, then turn chicken breast side up and continue roasting until internal temperature reaches 180.

Creating Your Own List

Obviously, you aren't going to shop for every single meal above – the list would be huge and you don't have time to cook a completely new meal every day at every meal time!

What we suggest is that you pluck the best sounding meals from the example days given above. If you have the same meal for lunch three or even five days in a row, for example, that's fine! All Ignite breakfasts are interchangeable with other Ignite breakfasts, lunches with lunches, and so on.

Whatever is convenient, satisfying, and works for you.

Make a list of the ingredients for your chosen meals, and then that becomes your personalized shopping list.

LAUNCH MEALS

DAY 1

Cereal and Fruit

Breakfast
7:00 AM

rice chex cereal, gluten free	2 Cup(s)
coconut milk beverage, unsweetened	1 1/2 Cup(s)
grapefruit	1 fruit

Greek Chicken Salad

Lunch
12:00 PM

romaine lettuce	1 Cup(s)
tomatoes	1/4 cup cherry tomatoes
drinking water	2 Cup(s)
extra virgin olive oil	1/2 Tbsp
cucumber	1/2 cucumber
feta cheese	1/4 cup, crumbled
chicken breast, cooked	2 oz

Cheese and Crackers

Snack
3:00 PM

cheese swiss	2 slice (1 oz)
brown rice crackers, no salt	6 crackers

Steak and Veggies

Dinner
6:00 PM

drinking water	2 Cup(s)
extra virgin olive oil	1 Tbsp
brussels sprouts, no salt, boiled	1 Cup(s)
black eyed peas	1/2 Cup(s)
beef top sirloin, lean, broiled	4 oz

DAY 2

Berry Overnight Oats
(recipe pg. 29)

Breakfast
7:00 AM

plain greek yogurt, nonfat	1 container
berry overnight oats	1 serving

Tilapia and Sweet Potato

Lunch
12:00 PM

extra virgin olive oil	1 Tbsp
drinking water	2 Cup(s)
sweet potato, no salt, baked	1/2 Cup(s)
tilapia fillets by sea best	4 oz
lemon juice	1 1 wedge

Quick Snack

Snack
3:00 PM

egg, hard boiled	1 large
drinking water	2 Cup(s)
pears	1 large

Mexican Dinner Bowls (Launch version)

Dinner
6:00 PM

romaine lettuce	2 Cup(s)
ground turkey, cooked	4 oz
tomatoes	1 medium
salsa, ready to serve	2 Tbsp
sweet corn kernels, no salt, boiled	1/4 Cup(s)
sour cream light	1 tablespoons

DAY 3

Breakfast Parfait

Breakfast
7:00 AM

drinking water	2 Cup(s)	0 cal
blueberries	1/2 Cup(s)	41 cal
plain greek yogurt, nonfat	1 container	100 cal
sunflower flax bread	1/2 slice	68 cal
almond butter, no salt	1/2 Tbsp	49 cal

Japanese Chicken Salad

Lunch
12:00 PM

drinking water	2 Cup(s)
romaine lettuce	2 Cup(s)
extra virgin olive oil	1/2 Tbsp
edamame soybeans, shelled	1/4 Cup(s)
tomatoes	1/2 cup cherry tomatoes
lemon juice	2 Tbsp
chicken breast, boneless skinless	4 oz
buckwheat groats, cooked	1 Cup(s)

Fruit and Nuts

Snack
3:00 PM

drinking water	2 Cup(s)
walnuts	1/4 cup shelled
oranges	1 fruit

Pork Tenderloin

Dinner
6:00 PM

drinking water	2 Cup(s)
pork tenderloin, lean, cooked	6 oz
zucchini/summer squash	2 cup, sliced
garlic	1 clove
olive oil	1 Tbsp

DAY 4

Blueberry Banana Shake

Breakfast
7:00 AM

blueberries	1 Cup(s)
drinking water	2 Cup(s)
bananas	1/2 medium
whey protein powder	1 Scoop
coconut milk beverage, unsweetened	1 1/2 Cup(s)

Fish Tacos

Lunch
12:00 PM

romaine lettuce	1 Cup(s)
extra virgin olive oil	1/2 Tbsp
tomatoes	1/2 cup cherry tomatoes
tilapia fillets by sea best	6 oz
yellow corn tortillas	2 tortillas
salsa, ready to serve	2 Tbsp

Afternoon Crunch

Snack
3:00 PM

drinking water	2 Cup(s)
plain greek yogurt, nonfat	1 container
seeds chia dried	1 oz
almonds	10 almond

Salmon and Veggies

Dinner
6:00 PM

salmon, cooked	4 oz
brussels sprouts, no salt, boiled	1/2 Cup(s)
beets	1 Cup(s)
black eyed peas	1/2 Cup(s)
coconut vegetable oil	1 Tbsp

DAY 5

Stuffed Breakfast Peppers
(recipe pg. 30)

Breakfast — 7:00 AM

drinking water	2 Cup(s)
breakfast stuffed peppers	1 serving
sunflower flax bread	1 slice
nectarines	1 fruit

Chicken Salad

Lunch — 12:00 PM

drinking water	2 Cup(s)
tomatoes	1/4 cup cherry tomatoes
romaine lettuce	1 Cup(s)
chicken breast, boneless skinless	4 oz
red peppers	1/2 medium
olive oil	1 Tbsp

Chocolate!

Snack — 3:00 PM

drinking water	2 Cup(s)
almonds	1/8 oz
dark chocolate bar	1/2 bar 1.45 oz

Shrimp and Greens

Dinner — 6:00 PM

shrimp, cooked	4 oz
edamame soybeans, shelled	1 Cup(s)
extra virgin olive oil	2 Tbsp
brussels sprouts, no salt, boiled	1 Cup(s)

DAY 6

Power Breakfast

Breakfast
7:00 AM

drinking water	2 Cup(s)
blueberries	1/2 Cup(s)
plain greek yogurt, nonfat	1 container
rice chex cereal, gluten free	1 Cup(s)
seeds flaxseed	1 tbsp, whole

Chicken Fiesta Salad
(recipe pg. 30)

Lunch
12:00 PM

drinking water	2 Cup(s)
chicken fiesta salad	1 serving

Cheese and Crackers

Snack
3:00 PM

pears	1 large
cheese swiss	1 slice (1 oz)
brown rice crackers, no salt	6 crackers

Beef and Broccoli

Dinner
6:00 PM

drinking water	2 Cup(s)
extra virgin olive oil	1/2 Tbsp
beef top sirloin, lean, broiled	4 oz
broccoli, no salt, steamed	2 Cup(s)

DAY 7

Eggs, Toast, and Jam

Breakfast
7:00 AM

egg, hard boiled	1 large
drinking water	2 Cup(s)
splenda sugar free strawberry jam preserves by smu...	1 Tbsp
ezekiel 4:9 sprouted 100% whole grain bread by foo...	2 slice

Tempeh Turkey

Lunch
12:00 PM

drinking water	2 Cup(s)
extra virgin olive oil	1 Tbsp
tempeh	2 oz
sweet potato, no salt, baked	1 medium
brussels sprouts, no salt, boiled	1 Cup(s)
ground turkey, cooked	4 oz

Almonds

Snack
3:00 PM

almonds	20 almond

Chicken Caesar

Dinner
6:00 PM

drinking water	2 Cup(s)
chicken breast, boneless skinless	4 oz
caeser dressing by great value	1 1/2 Tbsp
romaine lettuce	4 Cup(s)
lower sodium bacon by giant	2 slices
cherry tomatoes	5 tomatoes

2 Servings

berry overnight oats

Ingredients

oats	1/2 Cup(s)
plain greek yogurt, nonfat	4 oz
seeds flaxseed	1 tsp, whole
strawberries	1/2 Cup(s)
blueberries	1/2 Cup(s)
honey	1 Tbsp
skim milk with calcium	1/2 Cup(s)

Instructions

1. In a large glass jar or container, add oats and pour in milk.
2. Layer Greek yogurt, flax seeds and berries.
3. Refrigerate overnight and drizzle with honey before serving.

4 Servings

breakfast stuffed peppers

Ingredients

red peppers	2 medium
egg	4 egg
mushrooms	1/2 cup, pieces or slices
onions	1/2 medium
garlic	2 clove
fresh spinach	2 Cup(s)
tomatoes	1 medium
extra virgin olive oil	1 Tbsp
kosher salt	1/8 tsp
black pepper	1/4 tsp
cheese swiss	2 oz

Instructions

1. Preheat your oven to 375 degrees F.
2. Add olive oil to a medium sized skillet placed over a medium-heat.
3. Sauté onions and garlic until tender. Add in mushrooms, tomatoes and spinach. Cook until spinach is wilted.
4. Season to taste with salt and pepper. Turn off heat and set aside.
5. Cut two bell peppers in half and remove core/seeds. Place on baking sheet covered with foil.
6. In a small bowl whisk the 4 eggs until well beaten.
7. Divide the vegetable mixture equally among the bell pepper halves. Top each bell pepper with 1/4 of the beaten eggs.
8. Place the stuffed peppers in the oven and bake for 30 minutes. 9. Remove from oven and top each pepper with 0.5 oz of Swiss cheese. Place back in the oven for 10 minutes, or until cheese is melted and eggs are cooked through.

4 Servings

chicken fiesta salad

Ingredients

tomatoes	1 Cup(s)
romaine lettuce	4 Cup(s)
onions	1 medium
salsa, ready to serve	1/2 Cup(s)
sweet corn kernels, frozen	1 cup kernels
vegetable oil, palm	1 Tbsp
chicken breast skinless	16 oz
chicken fajita mix	1/2 pack
black beans, no salt, boiled	2 Cup(s)

Instructions

1. Rub chicken evenly with 1/2 the fajita seasoning. Heat the oil in a skillet over medium heat, and cook the chicken 8 minutes on each side, or until juices run clear; set aside.
2. In a large saucepan, mix beans, corn, salsa and other 1/2 of fajita seasoning. Heat over medium heat until warm.
3. Prepare the salad by tossing the greens, onion and tomato. Top salad with chicken and dress with the bean and corn mixture.

FAQS

Can I switch a meal on one day for another?

The answer is "Yes, but..."

On the meal plans you may switch meals relative to their specific sittings. In other words, you can switch the breakfast on Day 1 (Ginger Turmeric Smoothie) for the breakfast found on Day 3 (Avocado Egg Wrap) and so on. Lunches can be subbed out for other lunches and Dinners for other dinners found on your 7-Day Plan.

Here's the "but"...

You cannot take a dinner recipe and make it for lunch. Nor can you have "breakfast for dinner" and so on. The concepts of "nutrient timing", "energy balance" and "flavor pairing" outlined in the Main Book & Owner's Manual are infused into each and every meal in order to promote our 22-hour a day fat burning effect.

Bottom Line: Get creative, just not too creative

Swapping out foods

Although it's best to try and stick to the plan as best you can, we all need a little variety in our lives. If you are not a fan of a particular Angel Carb or veggie that you see on the meal plan, feel free to sub it out with another vegetable found on the list of Angel Carbs.

As a rule of thumb, try not to switch up the proteins (meat, fish, dairy etc.). However, I know we can't please everyone, so there are some exceptions to this rule based on preferences.

For example, if you absolutely cannot eat fish, then any white fish you see (e.g. tilapia, halibut, cod) may be substituted with chicken or turkey. If you do not eat or do not like to eat pork, it can be subbed with more calorically dense proteins like beef or salmon and vice versa.

Saving Time & Money

While eating healthily saves time and adds years to your life in the long run, it can add some dollars to your grocery bill right now, along with added prep time. With that in mind, here are a couple of tips that can knock dozens of dollars off your weekly grocery expenses while saving a ton of time as well.

Power Carbs

Pick one or two Power Carbs for the week to shop for and try to prep them in advance. Things like rice and quinoa are really inexpensive, plus they keep well in the refrigerator when prepped in larger amounts.

Prime Proteins

The largest expense on any meal plan are generally your protein selections so it's important to be conscious of not only how you choose, but how you prep as well.

To save time, I prep as much as possible each preparation session so I'm never left with the excuse that "I didn't have time" to make a meal. I also realize that nobody wants to eat a chicken breast on Friday that was made last Monday. With that said, at the start of the week I'll boil some eggs, grill a couple of chicken breasts and maybe some ground turkey. I'll also take that time to marinade or defrost some of the proteins that I know I'll have more time to make later on. This way you can count on your meats always staying fresh and not go to waste, while having the rest ready to cook when you need them.

Angel Carbs

The best way to save time and money when it comes to your veggies is to buy frozen. While fresh vegetables are obviously necessary in some dishes (salads etc.), frozen vegetables are half the price and are actually "fresher", due to the fact they are frozen immediately after picking.

Second, save some time by chopping your fresh vegetables at the start of the week and be sure to grab some fresh lemons while you're at the store. A squeeze of lemon on your chopped-up grab-and-go veggies will keep them fresher longer and prevent any browning.

Royal Fats

Buying your fat sources in bulk will be your biggest cost cutting measure by far. Things like nuts, oils, seeds, and butters last a long time and generally do not have to be refrigerated. Plus, while you are at the store a little cost comparison can go a long way; cashews are generally cheaper than almonds and walnuts, coconut oil is more expensive than olive oil, and almond butter is usually the cheapest of all the butters listed on your plan.

Our Top 10 Flavor Pairing & Weight Loss Combinations

Welcome to the most important piece of information you will find on your weight loss journey.

You won't find this in any of the other material and as you'll notice, I've sort of hidden this document near the end of this booklet.

The reason for placing this ultra-valuable list in "not-so-plain- sight" is because I want to reward those who have taken the time to read all of the material. Having a complete and clear understanding of ALL the material will not only fast-track you to your goal, but allow you to surpass that goal and hit other milestones for years to come.

These are the very same list of principles that my Cinderella research team extracted from the World's top bio-nutrition experts and expert-level scientists in my quest to help women like us lose the weight and keep it off forever in the healthiest and most efficient ways possible.

Even though most of these techniques are already built into the program itself, having them at your fingertips will give you the power to be even more flexible when it comes to food choices during the program and the knowledge needed to maintain the body that we build together over the next few weeks.

Enjoy!

1. Cinnamon & Starches/sugars

The evidence supporting Cinnamon's blood sugar regulating capabilities actually rival the power of prescription diabetes medication like Metphornin and Antagon.

Apart from the beneficial effects on insulin resistance, cinnamon can lower blood sugar by decreasing the amount of glucose that enters your bloodstream after a high-carb or sugar-rich meal by interfering with numerous digestive enzymes (this is a good thing), slowing down the breakdown of carbohydrates in your digestive tract.

Also, a compound in cinnamon can act on cells by mimicking insulin itself, therefore improving glucose uptake by your cells.

Numerous human studies have confirmed the anti-diabetic effects of cinnamon, showing that it can lower fasting blood sugar levels by 10–29%.

Put it in PLAY:

In order to get the benefits of the carbs you've been missing out on for so long while eliminating any option to store them as fat, try to add a pinch of cinnamon to all the meals that feature "Power Carbs" like fruit, potatoes rice etc.

Also do this prior to your cheat meals and if you have an episode where you fall off track with candy, cake, or any other sugary indulgence try to get a glass of hot water with cinnamon in you as soon as possible to regulate blood sugar and prevent all the sugar from ending up being stored as body fat in the places we desperately don't want it.

2. coffee and cocoa

This is by far one of the most powerful flavor-paring weapons you can use!

The regular consumption of cocoa controls fat-cell metabolism to reduce the absorption of fatty acids in your body. Besides aiding in reducing obesity, appropriate consumption of cocoa improves internal heat production (thermogenesis) in the liver and white adipose tissues.

Coffee on the other hand actually has the power to activate fat cells and mobilize them into your bloodstream to be used as energy.

This is why sprinkling a little cocoa powder in your coffee creates a supercharged fat- burning effect. While the cocoa has the ability to prevent the body from storing fat, the coffee helps free your fat cells to be burned faster.

Put it in PLAY:

In your morning coffee (free of fat-storing creams and milk) sprinkle in a pinch of pure cocoa powder to ramp up fat burning while preventing any fat accumulation.

Remember cocoa has a little caffeine in it as well so try not to consume this beverage after 1pm so you can get your beauty sleep.

3. carbs and protein

This is one of my favorites that I used every day on my own journey.

If you've been trying to lose weight, there is a good chance you have been shying away from carbs for the last couple years, which is why you may have been pleasantly surprised to see all the carbs on your menus and meal plans.

Although the meal planning is taken care of for you, it's important to know how to eat carbs to get all of their benefits while eliminating any of the unwanted negative effects, so I've gone into a little more detail on this one.

First, let's figure out why you should be eating more carbs....

If you've been shying away from carbs, just remember, Carbohydrates are your body's main source of energy: They help fuel your brain, kidneys, heart, muscles and central nervous system. For instance, fiber is a carbohydrate that aids in digestion, helps you feel full and keeps blood cholesterol levels in check. The way your meal plans are designed is to actually shuttle extra carbohydrates into your muscles and liver for energy rather than storing them as fat.

The truth is, a carbohydrate-deficient diet may cause headaches, fatigue, weakness, difficulty concentrating, nausea, constipation, bad breath and vitamin and mineral deficiencies.

The problem is that most of us pair our carbs with the wrong types of foods or with nothing at all. Whether you eat a bowl of healthy rice or smashed sweet potato that has zero added sugar, or you reach for a chocolate bar or candy that's loaded with extra sugar, your body goes through similar processes.

Within minutes your body spikes insulin to convert carbs into a form of sugar called glycogen that is used for energy. The problem is, the faster the conversion rate, the more likely those carbs are going to end up as fat rather than being used as energy.

The key here is to slow down your body's insulin response. This is already taken care of for you in the program by selecting the most fibrous carbs on the planet which cause an immediate slowdown. However, you can enhance this effect by including something that has the ability to manage blood sugar levels even more efficiently.

By adding healthy protein choices along with your power carbs, you increase your ability to prevent those carbs from getting stored as fat while increasing fat burning capabilities with the thermogenic effect of lean protein sources.

Put it in Play:

Remember, this is one of the key reasons why the Japanese are able to eat twice as many carbs as any other country, yet stay so lean and healthy. Again, this is taken care of for you throughout the program, but I want this drilled into you for when you're all done:

Never eat even healthy carbs by themselves.

Think toast and jam, fruit by itself, grilled cheese sandwiches. For example, if you're going to have a bowl of pasta, make sure there is a lean "Prime-Protein" in there like

chicken or even meatballs. If mashed potatoes are on the menu be sure there is a side of salmon, for example. Don't worry about the increased calories from the protein – think about those extra calories as insulin-spike-reducing, fat-accumulation-preventing nutrients that help you get leaner by actually eating more food.

4. lemon and apple cider vinegar

It seems like apple cider vinegar (ACV) and lemon detoxes have been the "darling" of internet cleanses over the last few years and there's good reason for it. When you list the proven detoxification benefits of both, you end up with a duo that will have your insides looking and feeling on point.

The problem with those 1, 3- and 5-day cleanses are not only that they have you guzzling gallons of lemon juice and ACV, but they inevitably come to an end. There are no directions for including them into your daily routine and almost more importantly, they never list all their other benefits including their ability to increase insulin sensitivity, mobilize fatty tissue for energy and enhanced mood and cognitive function.

Here's how it works:

ACV and lemons are high in potassium and acetic acid which stimulate brain and nerve function. When these two functions are not at their peak, you are more likely to cave into cravings.

The brain's key decision maker, the Pre-Frontal Cortex thrives when flooded with potassium which allows you to keep willpower functioning at optimal levels. Also, multiple studies have shown your intestinal lining is left spotless from the ACV's acetic acid, and as a result, people show better mood and decision making because of an improved "brain-gut" connection.

Combine all this with a boost in energy, craving suppression, and heart health and from the pectin found in the lemons and the chlorogenic acid in the vinegar and you can never go wrong with this dynamic duo.

Although the two do produce an amplified synergistic effect when taken together, there is no reason you can't find a few ways to squeeze them in on their own separately, which we'll look at now.

Put it in Play:

Try to include lemon into any meal you see fit. That means on fish, potatoes, rice and as a salad dressing base. Squeeze some into your water whenever you can to ramp-up taste and keep a steady stream of brain-enhancing, craving-reducing nutrients flowing all day long.

Lemon juice and ACV help to suppress your appetite and aids in digestion and alkalinity as well. By helping you feel fuller longer, you end up overeating less.

Studies have shown that if you maintain a more alkaline diet you will lose weight faster, so do your best to use ACV as a base for the salad dressings that list vinegar as its base or even as a marinade base for some of your meats.

Finally, you can get this duo in you the most efficient way by adding a tiny dose to your water throughout the day.

A few years ago, I wanted to see if I could stop drinking (and spending a ton of money) on coffee. When I dropped the coffee, I added ACV and lemon to the giant bottle of water that I promised myself I'd drink each day on my coffee detox.

After a few days I not only noticed improvement in mood and sleep, but I maintained consistent energy levels throughout the day without the coffee-crash!

5. turmeric and honey

While many of our flavor pairing rituals have been borrowed from the Japanese, this particular little gem is one that the Japanese borrowed from India. At first this may seem like an unusual pairing, and you're right, it is - but once you find out the benefits of this powerful combination, you'll see why it made the list.

First turmeric on its own has been touted recently as one of the new miracle foods that the health and wellness community has latched onto over the last few years as a key anti-inflammatory miracle food. Since inflammation is not only related to increased rates of cancer, obesity, heart attack and especially brain related disease like dementia and Alzheimer's, it's no wonder everyone is telling you to take it.

However, there is something that they're forgetting to tell you. While turmeric in its root and powder form on its own is very effective for digestive purposes, most promote turmeric itself as a key anti-inflammatory aid. The problem is and what they don't tell you is that the active ingredient needed to reduce inflammation, curcumin gets lost along the way. The most powerful part of this whole equation, the curcumin, cannot cross the barrier needed to be absorbed by your blood, and thus most of us never get the cure-all effects!

What you need in order to get all the weight loss, anti-inflammatory and life- lengthening effects is a little piperine and a controlled insulin bump - not a spike - just a little bump.

Put it in play

In order to get all the benefits of curcumin via the aforementioned delivery system (piperine and increased insulin release) the answer is simple and delicious.

The way most Cinderella Success Stories make this happen is by having a mid-day soothing Turmeric-Pepper-Honey Tea. Although it may not sound super tasty, I'm sure you'll have no problem adding it to your daily routine after just one cup. The honey will add the tiny insulin release needed to absorb the curcumin and the piperine will act almost like a key unlocking the piperine from the turmeric.

Instructions:

- Steep or boil 1 cup of water
- Add ½ teaspoon of turmeric powder
- 1 pinch of black pepper (preferably fresh ground)
- ½ tsp. honey

6. fiber and carbohydrates

Are you filling up on fiber? If you are looking to lose weight while still enjoying the carbs you love, you should be!

Including high-fiber foods in your diet is a healthy and natural way to both lose weight while helping to reduce high blood sugar. As an added incentive, you'll be able to stay full longer, which is also going to help you knock off a couple of bonus pounds as well.

Eating lots of fiber like the kinds found in your "Angel Carbs", as well as the starchy carbs like rice and potatoes etc. found at the top of the "Power Carbs" list, helps eliminate fat all over the body and specifically the deadly "visceral fat" that surrounds most of our organs!

Finally, if that wasn't enough, fiber promotes excellent bowel health, lowers the risk of cancer and heart disease, while also controlling your blood sugar.

When fiber is digested, your body handles it differently than the way in which refined carbohydrates, such as white flour, are digested. A portion of the fiber simply passes through your digestive system intact. This difference means that eating foods rich in fiber eliminates any dramatic spikes in high blood sugar because fiber doesn't require insulin to digest, which also means that it can be counted against the total carbohydrates of that particular meal.

When you look at a nutrition facts table, you will typically find the suggested serving size at the top of the table and the grams of total carbohydrates per serving lower in the table.

Below the total carbs, you will see the fiber content listed in grams. Fiber is accounted for as part of the total carbohydrates found in a food. In other words, it's listed twice - once in the listing under "fiber" and once as part of the total carbohydrate count, which also includes starches and sugars.

For example, if a bowl of oatmeal has 30 grams of carbs but has 15 grams of fiber, you are only left with 15 total carbs that impact the body!

Put it in Play

Now, I've already given you recommendations on portion sizes and as I always say, I never want you to be a slave to calorie counting, so I've taken care of a lot of this for you. All of your Power Carbs, specifically the top 10 on the list, are chock-full of fiber.

And in those higher carbohydrate meals I always recommended that you load up on Angel Carbs because they are also fiber-rich, which will help with our goal of reducing total impact carbs.

However, this is real life and I know that sometimes you're not going to be able to eat exactly what's on the Cinderella Menu...

So, if you're out and about – or even when you're getting groceries, have a look at your labels.

If you are absolutely DYING for carbs, have a look at the label of the food you choose and look at the carb vs fiber amounts.

If it's a higher carb option like a granola bar you won't feel guilty when you see that the fiber content is almost equal to the carbohydrates!

That means you can sometimes have your cake and eat it too (as long as that cake has some fiber in it).**zinc and waking up**

That's right! One part of this equation is extremely easy – all you have to do is open those eyes and get your butt out of bed... the other part, the zinc part, isn't so simple... it's not hard, but it's not simple either.

Zinc is a trace element that is absolutely essential for a healthy immune system. A lack of zinc can make a person more susceptible to disease and illness. This powerful little mineral is responsible for a number of functions in the human body, and it helps stimulate the activity of at least 100 different enzymes. The good news is that only a small intake of zinc is necessary to reap the benefits.

The bad news is that even getting a small amount of zinc in our body is a tough task. Most foods are low in zinc and most high-level zinc foods are also high carb foods as well - not that that's a bad thing, but in order to get the necessary amount of zinc needed to facilitate weight loss, immune function and better sleep, you'd have to be eating a lot of carbs very often.

However, eggs have absolutely zero carbs and a large amount of zinc, so they are an excellent choice.

Put it in play

As you'll see, we've already taken care of this for you in your meal plans by adding many meals that include eggs in one way or another. Whether it be as a baking ingredient in your lunches, dinners, and snacks, or in the more traditional forms of just having eggs for breakfast.

Not a fan of eggs? I'm with you! I never really was either and sometimes busy ladies like us don't have time to whip up eggs every morning.

If you're in that category, I've included the most naturally zinc rich foods in all of your morning meals and if you're in a hurry, they're in those shakes too. Plus, most fitness gurus recommend taking the best part out of the egg, the yolk, which happens to be the part of the egg that contains all the zinc. Once you have a look at some of the recipes provided, I think you'll agree that eggs are a pleasant tasting and nutritious way to start the day.

And if you're worried about cholesterol, the team has portioned out servings so that you are only getting the newly proven, doctor recommended, heart-healthy serving of healthy cholesterol.

7. olive oil and salt

While both salt and olive oil make a welcome addition to almost any meal, I'm not talking about a flavor pairing you put in your mouth here. Of all places, I actually want these 2 health and wellness powerhouses in your tub! Out of all the pairings and combinations listed, this one definitely ranks in my top 3 - not only for the proven scientific and biological benefits, but for the way it makes me feel... almost immediately!

Let's get the "science-stuff" out of the way first.

Extra Virgin Olive Oil itself contains vitamin E, anti-oxidants, and compounds such as squalene and oleocanthal, which prevent aging and repair skin damage. Olive oil is non- toxic, anti-microbial, and hypoallergenic.

Plus, on top of that this is what the beautiful Sophia Lauren attributes to be the sole reason for her almost ageless existence. When asked how she stays looking so young well into her 80's she said: "my mother and sisters all looked old before their time, the only thing I did differently was something a friend's grandmother showed me in my teenage years. Whenever I draw a bath, I release one cap of olive oil into the water".

As for the second half of the equation, salt. When adding it to your bath, most women prefer the Epsom Salt variety for its increased mineral properties, of which there are 21 to be exact. These include magnesium, potassium, sodium, sulfur, zinc, calcium, chloride, iodide, and bromide, all of which work synergistically to nourish our bodies.

When it comes to weight loss specifically this combination adds a double-punch by adding a dual pulling effect drawing the toxins from the body that induce inflammation and prevent fat mobilization for energy. This itself leads to 3 other key benefits:

1) Reduce insomnia by increasing circulation and adding magnesium, a common ingredient in most sleep-aids
2) Relief of arthritis pain including osteoarthritis, rheumatoid arthritis, and psoriatic arthritis.
3) Improving skin quality and relief from eczema.

In one German study, patients with active eczema soaked one arm in a dead sea salt solution and their other arm in tap water for 15 minutes a day for 6 weeks. Soaking in the Dead Sea salt solution significantly improved skin barrier function, hydration, and inflammation compared with the tap water-treated side.

Put it in Play:

Simply add 1 capful of olive oil and as much as one cup of Epsom salts to your warm bath. The more is better approach is NOT recommended here unless you want to step out of that bath feeling like a pork-chop ready for the grill!

And even with this minimal dose of each, be sure to towel off thoroughly. For the sake of anybody else who lives with you, maybe devote a special towel to your salty-oil bath as well.

Don't have time for a bath? Yes, you do.

I hate to be one of those people who say "make time" but... MAKE TIME.

Light a candle, draw the bath, put in your "potion" and turn everything (and everyone) else off.

This is your time, do something for you and relax. Speaking of relaxing, I almost forgot to mention... remember the whole increased cortisol/stress thing keeping us ladies chubby?

A 10-minute warm bath (with or without salt and oil) has been proven to reduce blood pressure by 10% and cortisol levels by 20.

Bottom Line... make time for yourself, and your bath!

8. ginger and orange

As complex and as efficient as the human body is, performing literally a million tasks at once, it still hasn't figured out how to do everything really well all at once. What I mean is, your body kind of has a "one track mind' and if it is caught up doing one large task, some of the others will suffer - especially when it comes to digestion.

Think of digestion as a workout for the entire inside of your body...

... Stomach acids are mobilized to break down food, the liver and kidneys jump in to eliminate toxins, all while a few liters of blood are devoted to fueling the whole process.

For many of us, our digestive system has been experiencing an all-day traffic jam, even after the smallest meals, which is one of the primary reasons most women have trouble losing weight or keeping it off. If the body is caught up with digesting and breaking down food, it cannot focus on our primary goal over the next few weeks of fat elimination and creating hormonal balance.

The ginger portion of this equation was lifted from our go-to healthy country, Japan, who eat ginger with almost every meal in its pickled form, while the citrus half was taken from the Germans who typically try to add oranges to almost each and every heavy meal.

This little root contains nine different substances that have been found to stimulate serotonin receptors in the gut, which provide benefits to the gastrointestinal system, reducing gut-related inflammation and enhancing nutrient absorption.

Ginger is classified as a carminative (reducing intestinal gas) and an intestinal spasmolytic (soothes the intestinal tract), while inducing gut motility. Additionally, it helps aid in the production of bile, making it particularly helpful in digesting fats.

The other half of this equation, the citrus (specifically oranges), takes care of the rest. For many of us even if our digestion is on track we fail when it comes to the most important part, nutrient and mineral absorption. Getting your hormones to work together to mobilize fat as fuel takes a lot of help, or "ingredients", and oranges have everything we need.

While the heavy dose of vitamin C in any citrus fruit plays a key role in helping the gut and intestinal track absorb those precious nutrients, oranges perform best when it comes to assimilation of iron – a key fat mobilization and energy enhancing aid.

Oranges take multitasking to the next level by promoting a "blunted" insulin spike that

not only helps digest the food itself, but soothes insulin sensitivity as well.

Put it in Play:

Option 1 (my go-to)

Almost every night before bed I treat myself to an "Orange Ginger Digestive" tea so my body can focus on burning fat while I sleep instead of devoting all its energy to digesting my last meal. While you may be able to find an orange ginger tea at the grocery store, I prefer to make my own just because I know I'm getting about 5-10 times the nutrients needed with the DIY version.

To make enough for a few cups later in the week, or even better, a cold glass in the afternoon tomorrow, boil 4 cups of water with 1 inch of ginger sliced into tiny pieces along with one full orange sliced into circular slices. Add a natural sweetener if you like and let this powerful concoction go to work.

By the way, this is one of my favorite nighttime "craving-killers" as well!

9. oxygen & h20

This combination is designed to flood the body, blood and brain with the primary elements that keep you alive... makes sense that this would be beneficial, right?

We do this by ingesting massive doses of oxygen while reinvigorating its only means of transportation, your blood.

Again, cortisol and dehydration levels are naturally at their highest upon rising and in the mid-afternoon. Although you may not feel stressed or dehydrated when you wake up, your stress hormone is pumping in excess in order to get the rest of the body ready for action. And while you were snoozing, every cell went through a massive regeneration and renewal process, using a large amount of your body's water supply.

At around 1-3 in the afternoon, cortisol and dehydration reach their second peak. For most of us we've already dealt with a bunch of micro-stressors that could stem from a number of bothersome or annoying situations and in the midst of all this it's only natural that you haven't consumed the right amount of water to stay hydrated.

The bottom line is, if your stress hormone is pumping and you're dehydrated the last thing your body is focused on is losing weight.

In fact, the opposite is true; you're more likely to add pounds here as the body looks to save up fuel (fat and water) in case of emergency.

With all this in mind, it's time to use an easy, yet proven technique that immediately suppresses cortisol and stress levels along with a cocktail that provides natural energy, rehydration, and detoxification while alkalizing the body.

Put it in Play:

Ideally, every morning and every afternoon when you can, you will practice 10-20 reps of breathwork for immediate cortisol reduction plus all day cortisol regulation and to improve Tissue Function & Prevention.

All of our organs perform better when fully oxygenated, plus most diseases cannot thrive in an optimally oxygenized environment. As an added bonus, this will provide an immediate and prolonged stimulation of the lymphatic system too.

This routine should be followed by drinking 1-16oz (250ml-500ml) of "alkalized water", resulting in a 20-24% boost in metabolic function, and eliminating dehydration after 7-8 hours of sleep. You'll also increase nutrient absorption and create an "Alkaline" environment in your body that provides clean energy, fat oxidization and mental focus using some of the principles borrowed from flavor-pairing #4 (lemon and ACV).

Breathwork Technique

1 REP EQUALS:

- Take a deep breath in through the nose that lasts 4 seconds
- Hold your breath for two seconds
- Exhale from the nose and mouth "through the diaphragm" for 5-6 seconds releasing every last bit of air
- During these repetitions focus on nothing but your breathing. This may be tough to do at first. Thoughts will enter your mind but simply recognize that thought, dismiss it, and refocus again on your breathing.

X15-20 repetitions

Alkalized Water INGREDIENTS*:

WATER: 500ml/16.9 fl oz (minimum) LEMON JUICE: ½ squeezed lemon

This routine should be followed by drinking 1-16oz (250ml-500ml) of "alkalized water", resulting in a 20-24% boost in metabolic function, and eliminating dehydration after 7-8 hours of sleep. You'll also increase nutrient absorption and create an "Alkaline" environment in your body that provides clean energy, fat oxidization and mental focus using some of the principles borrowed from flavor-pairing #4 (lemon and ACV).

Breathwork Technique

1 REP EQUALS:

- Take a deep breath in through the nose that lasts 4 seconds
- Hold your breath for two seconds
- Exhale from the nose and mouth "through the diaphragm" for 5-6 seconds releasing every last bit of air
- During these repetitions focus on nothing but your breathing. This may be tough to do at first. Thoughts will enter your mind but simply recognize that thought, dismiss it, and refocus again on your breathing.

X15-20 repetitions

Alkalized Water INGREDIENTS*:

- WATER: 500ml/16.9 fl oz (minimum)

- LEMON JUICE: ½ squeezed lemon

This routine should be followed by drinking 1-16oz (250ml-500ml) of "alkalized water", resulting in a 20-24% boost in metabolic function, and eliminating dehydration after 7-8 hours of sleep. You'll also increase nutrient absorption and create an "Alkaline" environment in your body that provides clean energy, fat oxidization and mental focus using some of the principles borrowed from flavor-pairing #4 (lemon and ACV).

Breathwork Technique

1 REP EQUALS:

- Take a deep breath in through the nose that lasts 4 seconds
- Hold your breath for two seconds
- Exhale from the nose and mouth "through the diaphragm" for 5-6 seconds releasing every last bit of air
- During these repetitions focus on nothing but your breathing. This may be tough to do at first. Thoughts will enter your mind but simply recognize that thought, dismiss it, and refocus again on your breathing.

X15-20 repetitions

Alkalized Water INGREDIENTS*:

- WATER: 500ml/16.9 fl oz (minimum)
- LEMON JUICE: ½ squeezed lemon
- 1 pinch of baking soda or sea salt

FREE BONUS: The Cinderella Accelerator And The Movement Sequencing Guide

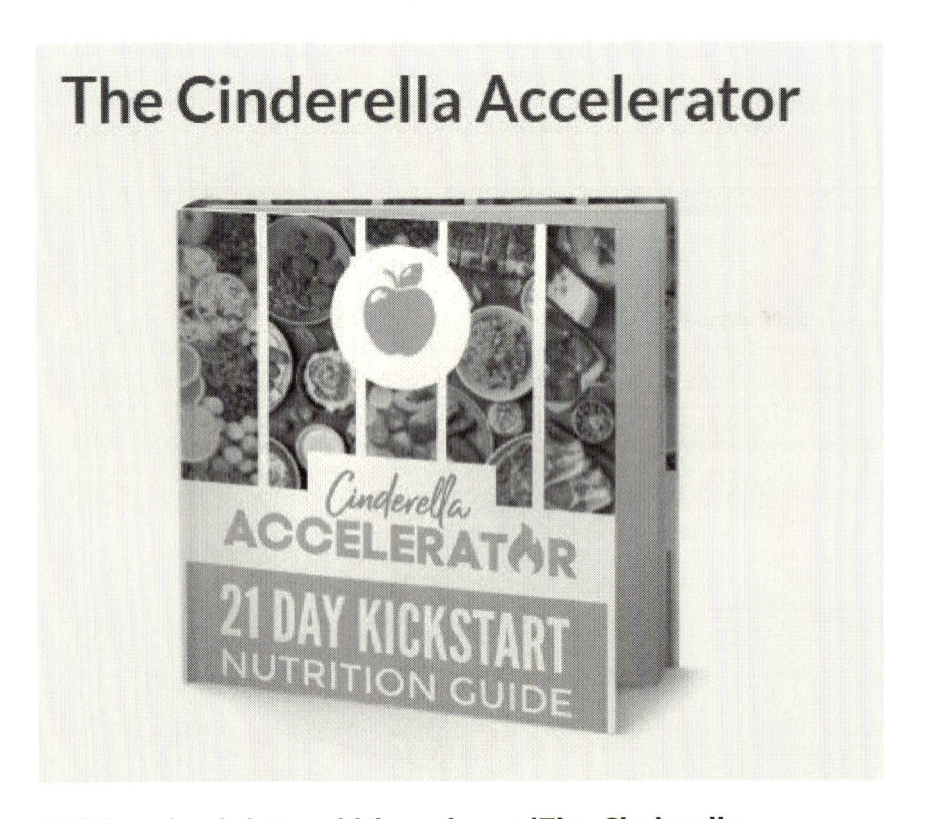

Pdf download: https://tinyurl.com/The-Cinderella-Accelerator

The Movement Sequencing Guide

Pdf download: https://tinyurl.com/The-Movement-Sequencing-Guide